Table of Contents

Introduction	4
Chapter 1	8
Introduction to Female Reproductive Health	8
Chapter 2	15
Understanding Ectopic Pregnancy	15
Chapter 3	24
Ovarian Cysts: Types, Symptoms, and Treatments	24
Chapter 4	32
Pelvic Organ Prolapse: What Every Woman Needs to Know	32
Chapter 5	42
Uterine Fibroids: Causes, Symptoms, and Management	42
Chapter 6	51
Endometrial Cancer: Early Detection and Treatment	51
Chapter 7	60
Premature Ovarian Failure: The Impact on Fertility	60
Chapter 8	69
Female Infertility: Causes and Solutions	69
Chapter 9	79
Introduction to Male Reproductive Health	79
Chapter 10	88
Prostatitis: Understanding Symptoms and Treatment	88
Chapter 11	96
Male Infertility: Identifying and Overcoming Challenges	96
Chapter 12	105
Introduction to STIs: Prevention and Awareness	105
Chapter 13	112
Genital Herpes: Myths, Facts, and Management	112
Chapter 14	120
Gonorrhea: Symptoms, Diagnosis, and Treatment	120

Chapter 15	127
The Psychological Impact of STIs	127
Chapter 16	135
Prevention and Safe Practices: A Guide to Protecting Reproductive Health	135
Chapter 17	143
Holistic Health Approaches to Reproductive Wellness	143
Chapter 18	152
The Role of Modern Medicine in Reproductive Health	152
Chapter 19	160
Lifestyle Choices and Reproductive Health	160
Chapter 20	168
Surgical Interventions: When Necessary	168
Chapter 21	176
Fertility Treatments and Assisted Reproductive Technologies (ART)	176
Chapter 22	185
The Future of Male and Female Infertility Treatments	185
Chapter 23	193
Genomic and Personalized Medicine in Reproductive Health	193
Chapter 24	201
Adolescent Reproductive Health	201
Chapter 25	208
Reproductive Health in Your 20s and 30s	208
Chapter 26	216
Reproductive Health in Your 40s and Beyond	216
Chapter 27	225
The Role of Partners in Reproductive Health	225
Chapter 28	232
Coping with Infertility: Emotional Support and Treatment	232
Chapter 29	239
Managing the Diagnosis of Reproductive Cancers	239
Chapter 30	246
Overcoming the Stigma of STIs	246
Chapter 31	254

Impact of Sexual Health on Mental Well-being 254
Chapter 32 262
Sexual Health Education: Empowering the Next Generation 262
Chapter 33 269
The Role of Healthcare Providers in Prevention 269
Chapter 34 276
Public Health Initiatives in Reproductive Health 276
A Call to Action for Better Reproductive and Sexual Health 284
Summary of Key Takeaways 284
References 289

Reproductive and Sexual Health: A Comprehensive Guide to Understanding, Managing, and Preventing Key Conditions

Introduction

Reproductive and sexual health is an essential aspect of overall well-being that directly impacts individuals' physical, emotional, and social lives. It encompasses a wide range of conditions that affect both men and women, each of which can have profound effects on health, relationships, and personal identity. From the challenges of fertility and sexual health to the emotional and physical toll of chronic conditions, the journey through reproductive health can be complex and multifaceted. Whether dealing with infertility, a sexually transmitted infection, or reproductive cancers, each individual's experience is unique, and the need for accurate, compassionate, and accessible information is vital.

This book seeks to provide a thorough and comprehensive understanding of common reproductive and sexual health conditions, helping individuals make informed decisions regarding prevention, diagnosis, treatment, and management. Our focus is on conditions that frequently affect both men and women, such as ectopic pregnancy, ovarian cysts, prostatitis, pelvic organ prolapse, endometrial cancer, male infertility, uterine fibroids, premature ovarian failure, genital herpes, and gonorrhea. Through this exploration, we aim to highlight the importance of proactive health management and the role of education in empowering individuals to take control of their reproductive and sexual health.

Each chapter of this book has been carefully crafted to provide an in-depth look at the various conditions that can impact reproductive and sexual health. We will examine the causes, risk factors, and symptoms of these conditions, ensuring that readers understand the complexities of each one. Additionally, we will delve into the various treatment options available, ranging from medical interventions to lifestyle changes, and explore how advancements in reproductive medicine have transformed the way these conditions are diagnosed and managed. Through this, we hope to empower individuals to make informed decisions about their health and navigate their experiences with confidence.

The impact of reproductive and sexual health conditions goes beyond the physical. Many of these conditions bring emotional and psychological challenges, such as feelings of frustration, isolation, and grief. Whether struggling with infertility, the emotional toll of chronic pelvic pain, or the stigma associated with sexually transmitted infections, the mental and emotional well-being of those affected should never be overlooked. This book emphasizes the importance of addressing the emotional side of reproductive health, encouraging individuals to seek support and to prioritize their mental health as they navigate these challenges.

Socially, reproductive health often carries a stigma, particularly when it comes to conditions like genital herpes, gonorrhea, and male infertility. These issues can sometimes feel isolating, with individuals facing judgment or misconceptions that further complicate their experience. Through this book, we aim to reduce this stigma by offering honest, factual information and encouraging open conversations about these often-taboo topics. By providing a safe and non-judgmental space for discussion, we hope to foster a greater sense of understanding and empathy, allowing individuals to feel more comfortable seeking care and support.

The goal of this book is not only to inform but also to equip individuals with the tools and knowledge needed to take proactive steps in maintaining and improving their reproductive and sexual health. We will explore various prevention strategies that can help reduce the risk of developing certain conditions, such as safe sex practices, lifestyle changes, and early detection through regular screenings. The importance of early intervention cannot be overstated, as many reproductive health conditions are more easily managed when detected early, leading to better outcomes and a higher quality of life.

Furthermore, we recognize that reproductive health is a lifelong journey. From adolescence to menopause, and from the challenges of fertility to the realities of aging, every stage of life brings its own set of concerns and considerations. This book takes a holistic approach to reproductive and sexual health, addressing the unique needs of individuals at different stages of life, from adolescence to adulthood, and even into post-menopause. We also acknowledge the diverse experiences of individuals across different cultural, socioeconomic, and sexual orientations, offering a broad perspective on how reproductive and sexual health issues are experienced and managed in various contexts.

We will also examine the role of healthcare providers in supporting reproductive health. A strong relationship between patients and their healthcare providers is crucial for effective management of reproductive health conditions. This book will provide guidance on how to advocate for oneself in medical settings, communicate openly with healthcare professionals, and navigate treatment options in a way that aligns with individual values and goals. We will also discuss the importance of mental health support and the role of counseling, therapy, and support groups in helping individuals cope with the emotional and psychological impacts of reproductive health challenges.

Lastly, the landscape of reproductive health is constantly evolving. Advancements in medical research, treatments, and technology offer new hope for individuals facing reproductive health challenges. Whether it's groundbreaking fertility treatments, the development of new medications, or innovations in sexual health education, these advancements continue to change the way we approach reproductive and sexual health. This book aims to stay up-to-date with the latest research and provide readers with the most current information available to ensure they are equipped to make the best choices for their health.

By the end of this book, readers will have a deeper understanding of the conditions that affect reproductive and sexual health, as well as the knowledge and resources to take an active role in their health journey. Whether you are dealing with a reproductive health issue yourself, supporting a loved one, or simply seeking to learn more about this important aspect of human health, this book is designed to be an invaluable resource. It is our hope that by providing clear, accessible, and scientifically backed information, we can help individuals achieve better health outcomes, reduce stigma, and foster a society that values and prioritizes reproductive and sexual health for all.

Chapter 1

Introduction to Female Reproductive Health

Overview of the Female Reproductive System

The female reproductive system is an intricate network of organs designed for the purpose of reproduction, but it also plays a significant role in overall health and well-being. The system is made up of internal and external organs, each with its distinct function, working together to enable conception, pregnancy, and childbirth. It is important to understand the structure, function, and health of the female reproductive system, as it influences many aspects of a woman's physical, emotional, and hormonal health throughout her life.

At its core, the female reproductive system is divided into two main parts: the internal reproductive organs and the external genitalia. These organs not only facilitate reproduction but also influence menstruation, hormone production, and sexual function.

Internal Organs:

1. **Ovaries:** The ovaries are two small, almond-shaped glands located on either side of the uterus. Their primary function is the production and release of eggs (ova) and the secretion of key reproductive hormones, including estrogen and progesterone. These hormones regulate the menstrual cycle, influence sexual desire, and play a role in pregnancy.

2. **Fallopian Tubes:** These are narrow tubes that connect the ovaries to the uterus. The fallopian tubes serve as the pathway through which eggs travel from the ovaries to the uterus. Fertilization typically occurs here when sperm meets the egg.

3. **Uterus:** The uterus is a muscular organ where a fertilized egg implants and grows during pregnancy. It has three primary layers: the endometrium (inner lining), the myometrium (muscular layer), and the perimetrium (outer layer). The endometrium thickens during the menstrual cycle in preparation for a potential pregnancy, and if fertilization does not occur, it sheds during menstruation.

4. **Cervix:** The cervix is the lower part of the uterus, connecting the uterus to the vaginal canal. It serves as a passageway for menstrual blood to exit the body and for sperm to enter during intercourse. The cervix also produces mucus that varies in consistency throughout the menstrual cycle, which helps in either preventing or facilitating sperm movement.

5. **Vagina:** The vagina is a muscular canal that connects the cervix to the external genitalia. It serves as the passage for menstrual blood and a conduit for sperm during intercourse. Additionally, the vagina provides the necessary structure for childbirth, allowing the passage of a baby during labor.

External Genitalia: The external genitalia, collectively known as the vulva, include the labia (outer and inner folds of skin), the clitoris (a small organ highly sensitive to touch), and the urethra (the tube through which urine is excreted). The vulva serves as a protective barrier for the internal reproductive organs and plays a role in sexual pleasure and arousal.

The intricate design of these organs reflects the body's remarkable ability to carry out reproduction, and each component plays a role in ensuring a healthy and functional reproductive system. It is essential to recognize that these organs are not isolated; their functions are deeply interconnected, and an imbalance or issue in one area can often affect the others.

Importance of Maintaining Reproductive Health

The significance of maintaining good reproductive health cannot be overstated. The health of the female reproductive system is integral to overall well-being, influencing a woman's physical, mental, and emotional health across different stages of life. Women's reproductive health impacts not only fertility and childbirth but also hormone balance, sexual health, and the prevention of various conditions that can affect the reproductive organs.

Hormonal Balance and Its Role in Health: The female reproductive system is governed by a complex interplay of hormones. Estrogen, progesterone, luteinizing hormone (LH), and follicle-stimulating hormone (FSH) are all crucial in regulating the menstrual cycle, ovulation, and pregnancy. Hormonal imbalances can lead to conditions such as polycystic ovary syndrome (PCOS), endometriosis, and irregular menstrual cycles, which may result in symptoms like excessive hair growth, weight gain, mood swings, and difficulty conceiving. Therefore, maintaining hormonal balance is key not only for reproductive health but also for mental health and general vitality.

Menstrual Health: A regular, healthy menstrual cycle is an indicator of a well-functioning reproductive system. Menstrual health reflects the body's ability to maintain hormonal balance and supports the understanding of a woman's fertility. Issues such as heavy or irregular periods, painful cramps, and premenstrual syndrome (PMS) can point to underlying conditions that require attention. In some cases, menstrual irregularities may signal more significant reproductive health issues, such as fibroids, ovarian cysts, or even cancer.

A healthy menstrual cycle also supports the proper functioning of the ovaries and uterus, helping to prepare the body for potential pregnancy. When the cycle is disrupted, the possibility of conception may be affected, making it important for women to understand their menstrual health as part of their overall reproductive wellness.

Fertility and Conception: Reproductive health plays a crucial role in fertility, which is the ability to conceive and carry a pregnancy. Fertility can be influenced by a variety of factors, including age, medical conditions, lifestyle, and environmental factors. Maintaining reproductive health helps optimize fertility, whether a woman is trying to conceive or avoid pregnancy. Conditions such as blocked fallopian tubes, low egg reserve, or hormonal imbalances can impair fertility, while maintaining a healthy diet, regular exercise, and managing stress are beneficial for improving fertility.

Understanding fertility and the factors that impact it can be empowering for women, helping them make informed decisions about family planning and pregnancy. In cases where fertility issues arise, seeking professional medical advice and possible interventions, such as assisted reproductive technologies, can be part of the solution.

Sexual Health and Wellness: The state of a woman's reproductive health is directly linked to her sexual health. Reproductive organs such as the vagina and cervix play a central role in sexual function, and any problems in these areas can lead to discomfort, pain during intercourse, or reduced libido. Conditions like vaginitis, pelvic floor disorders, and sexually transmitted infections (STIs) can have significant impacts on sexual health, causing both physical and emotional distress.

Furthermore, the experience of sexual pleasure is also influenced by the health of the reproductive system. For many women, sexual health is intertwined with emotional and psychological well-being, and maintaining a healthy reproductive system can foster better intimacy and sexual relationships. Issues such as vaginal dryness, low libido, or painful intercourse are often symptoms of broader reproductive health conditions, which can be addressed with medical care or lifestyle changes.

Prevention and Early Detection of Health Issues: Preventative care and early detection are key components of maintaining reproductive health. Regular gynecological exams, including Pap smears, pelvic exams, and breast exams, are crucial for identifying potential issues early. These screenings can detect abnormalities such as cervical dysplasia, fibroids, or signs of infection before they become serious problems. Early intervention increases the chances of successful treatment and can help prevent further complications that may affect a woman's ability to conceive or carry a pregnancy to term.

Preventative measures also extend to lifestyle choices, including diet, exercise, and safe sexual practices. Maintaining a balanced diet rich in nutrients, such as folic acid, calcium, and iron, contributes to overall reproductive health. Regular physical activity helps regulate hormone levels and promotes better circulation, which is essential for healthy reproductive organs. Additionally, practicing safe sex and using protection to prevent STIs reduces the risk of infections that could compromise fertility and overall reproductive health.

The Role of Mental and Emotional Health: A woman's emotional and mental health is an often-overlooked aspect of reproductive health. Conditions such as infertility, miscarriage, or reproductive health disorders can take a significant emotional toll. Anxiety, depression, and stress can exacerbate physical symptoms and hinder recovery. On the other hand, mental well-being plays an important role in maintaining hormonal balance, regulating the menstrual cycle, and enhancing overall health.

Women experiencing reproductive health challenges should be encouraged to seek not only medical treatment but also psychological support. Counseling, therapy, and support groups can help manage the emotional aspects of reproductive health conditions, helping women cope with the stress, grief, and frustration that may accompany them.

The Importance of Reproductive Health Across Life Stages: The importance of maintaining reproductive health extends throughout a woman's life. From puberty through menopause, each stage of a woman's reproductive journey presents its own unique challenges and changes. The transition from adolescence to adulthood, the reproductive years, and the changes that occur during perimenopause and menopause require ongoing attention to the health of the reproductive system. Understanding the physical changes and managing them effectively ensures that women can live healthier lives at every stage.

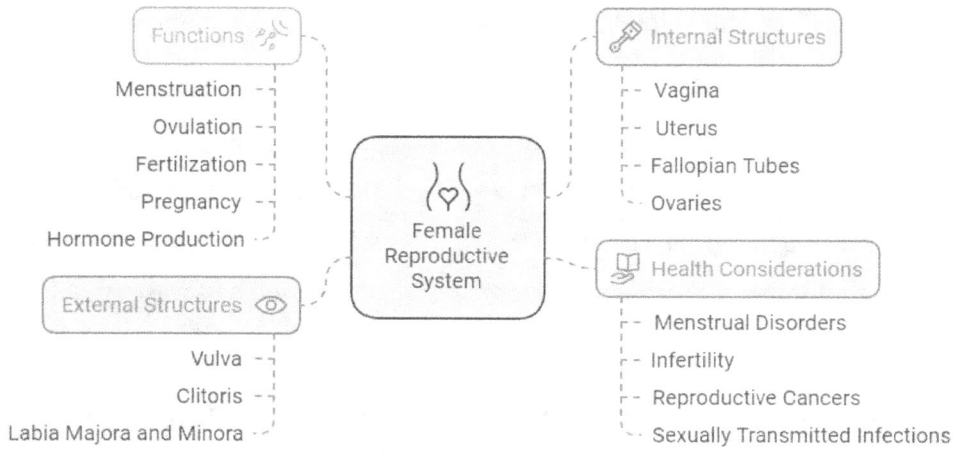

Conclusion

The female reproductive system is a remarkable and complex system that serves critical functions related to fertility, sexual health, and overall well-being. Understanding the importance of reproductive health, recognizing potential issues, and taking steps to maintain or restore it is essential for every woman. From hormonal balance to sexual wellness, regular screenings to lifestyle modifications, reproductive health is an integral part of every woman's life. By fostering a proactive approach to health and embracing preventive care, women can ensure that their reproductive system continues to function optimally, supporting their overall physical, emotional, and social well-being.

Chapter 2

Understanding Ectopic Pregnancy

An ectopic pregnancy occurs when a fertilized egg implants and grows outside the uterus, typically in one of the fallopian tubes. This condition is also known as a tubal pregnancy, but it can occur in other areas, such as the ovaries, cervix, or abdominal cavity. An ectopic pregnancy is a serious and potentially life-threatening condition that requires immediate medical attention. Unlike a normal pregnancy, which progresses within the protective environment of the uterus, an ectopic pregnancy cannot sustain a developing embryo, and if left untreated, can lead to severe complications for the mother.

Although the vast majority of pregnancies occur inside the uterus, ectopic pregnancies are relatively common, with approximately 1 in 50 pregnancies in the United States being ectopic. Understanding the causes, risk factors, symptoms, diagnosis, and treatment options for ectopic pregnancy is essential for early detection and management, which can prevent dangerous complications, such as internal bleeding, infertility, or even death.

Causes and Risk Factors of Ectopic Pregnancy

An ectopic pregnancy arises when a fertilized egg, instead of traveling into the uterus, becomes implanted in an area where it cannot develop normally. There are several causes and risk factors that can increase the likelihood of an ectopic pregnancy, many of which involve conditions or factors that affect the fallopian tubes or the transportation of the fertilized egg.

1. Damage or Abnormalities in the Fallopian Tubes: The most common cause of ectopic pregnancy is damage or blockage in the fallopian tubes, which can prevent the fertilized egg from moving properly into the uterus. Several conditions can affect the fallopian tubes, including:

- **Pelvic Inflammatory Disease (PID):** PID, often caused by sexually transmitted infections (STIs) such as chlamydia or gonorrhea, can lead to inflammation and scarring of the fallopian tubes, increasing the risk of an ectopic pregnancy.

- **Previous Surgery:** Past surgeries, such as tubal ligation (permanent contraception) or surgery for an ectopic pregnancy, can cause scarring or damage to the fallopian tubes, making it more difficult for a fertilized egg to travel through them.

- **Endometriosis:** This condition, in which tissue similar to the uterine lining grows outside the uterus, can cause pelvic adhesions or blockages in the fallopian tubes, increasing the risk of ectopic pregnancy.

2. History of Ectopic Pregnancy: Women who have had one ectopic pregnancy are at a higher risk of experiencing another in subsequent pregnancies. This is due to potential scarring or damage to the fallopian tubes, which may hinder the movement of eggs from the ovaries to the uterus.

3. Fertility Treatments: Certain fertility treatments, such as in vitro fertilization (IVF) or the use of fertility drugs that stimulate ovulation, can increase the risk of ectopic pregnancy. While IVF typically involves implanting the fertilized embryo directly into the uterus, complications from assisted reproductive techniques can sometimes cause embryos to implant in the fallopian tubes.

4. Use of Contraceptives: Although rare, women who use intrauterine devices (IUDs) or the contraceptive injection may have an increased risk of ectopic pregnancy. These methods of contraception are highly effective at preventing pregnancy, but if conception does occur, the risk of an ectopic pregnancy is higher.

5. Smoking and Age: Women who smoke are more likely to experience tubal damage and have a higher risk of ectopic pregnancy. Smoking can interfere with the function of the fallopian tubes and reduce the effectiveness of the cilia (hair-like structures) that help move the fertilized egg toward the uterus. Additionally, women over the age of 35 may be at an increased risk of ectopic pregnancy due to natural age-related changes in fertility and an increased likelihood of fallopian tube abnormalities.

6. Other Factors: Other potential risk factors for ectopic pregnancy include:

- **Multiple sexual partners:** This increases the likelihood of STIs, which can cause PID and lead to tubal damage.
- **Douching:** This practice can disrupt the natural balance of bacteria in the vagina and may increase the risk of infection, potentially leading to pelvic inflammatory disease.

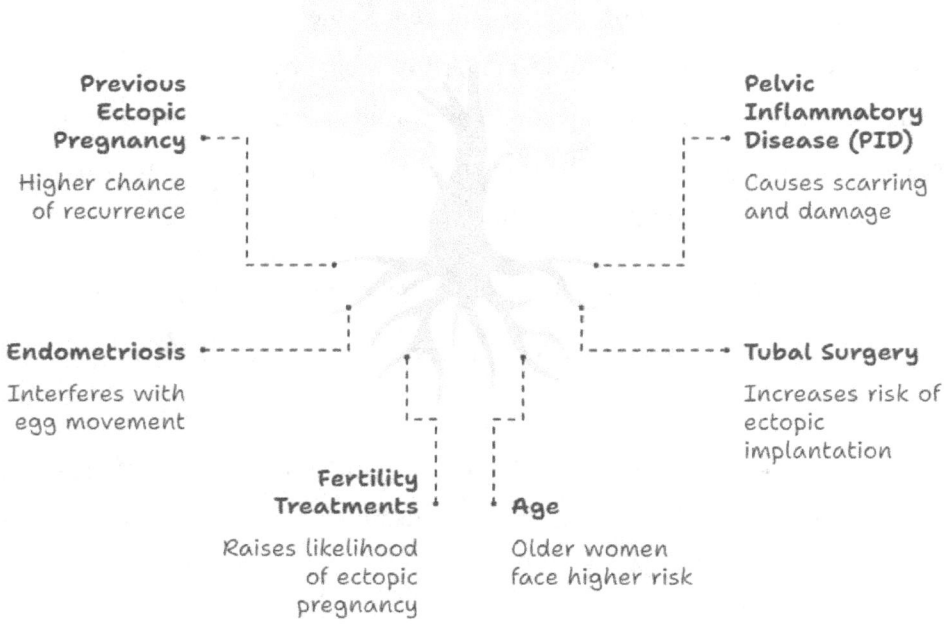

Symptoms and Diagnosis of Ectopic Pregnancy

Recognizing the symptoms of an ectopic pregnancy is crucial for prompt diagnosis and treatment. Ectopic pregnancies do not always cause symptoms in the early stages, which is why regular prenatal care and early monitoring are essential. As the pregnancy progresses, however, symptoms typically become more noticeable.

Common Symptoms

1. **Abdominal Pain or Discomfort:** Pain is the most common symptom of an ectopic pregnancy. The pain may start as mild and intermittent, often felt on one side of the abdomen, and may become more severe as the pregnancy progresses. As the fertilized egg grows and causes the fallopian tube to stretch, the pain can become sharp and localized. In some cases, the pain may also radiate to the shoulder or neck due to internal bleeding irritating the diaphragm.

2. **Vaginal Bleeding:** Spotting or light bleeding can occur with an ectopic pregnancy, often mistaken for a normal menstrual period. The bleeding may be lighter or heavier than usual, and it may be associated with abdominal pain. In some cases, the bleeding may be dark brown or watery.

3. **Shoulder Pain:** Shoulder pain is a significant red flag for an ectopic pregnancy. If the fallopian tube ruptures, blood may pool in the abdomen and irritate the diaphragm, leading to shoulder pain. This symptom often occurs along with other signs of internal bleeding and should be treated as an emergency.

4. **Dizziness or Fainting:** As an ectopic pregnancy progresses and leads to rupture, significant internal bleeding can occur. This can cause a drop in blood pressure, leading to dizziness, lightheadedness, or fainting.

5. **Nausea and Vomiting:** While nausea is common in early pregnancy, it can also occur with ectopic pregnancies. However, in the case of ectopic pregnancy, the nausea may be accompanied by more severe pain and bleeding.

Diagnostic Methods

To confirm an ectopic pregnancy, healthcare providers rely on a combination of physical examinations, blood tests, and imaging techniques.

1. **Pelvic Exam:** During a pelvic exam, a healthcare provider may be able to detect tenderness or swelling in the pelvic area, which can suggest an ectopic pregnancy.
2. **Blood Tests:** A blood test to measure levels of human chorionic gonadotropin (hCG) is essential for diagnosing pregnancy. In a typical pregnancy, hCG levels double every 48 hours. In an ectopic pregnancy, the hCG levels may rise more slowly or plateau, which is a key indicator that the pregnancy is not developing normally.
3. **Ultrasound:** A transvaginal ultrasound is the most effective imaging technique used to diagnose an ectopic pregnancy. This allows doctors to examine the uterus, fallopian tubes, and other pelvic structures to determine if the pregnancy is located outside of the uterus.

If an ectopic pregnancy is suspected, it is critical to seek medical attention immediately. Delaying diagnosis and treatment can lead to dangerous complications.

Treatment Options and Complications

Once an ectopic pregnancy is diagnosed, treatment is necessary to prevent the serious complications that can arise. The goal of treatment is to remove or stop the development of the ectopic pregnancy while preserving the health and fertility of the woman.

1. Medical Treatment: In early-stage ectopic pregnancies, medication may be used to stop the growth of the fertilized egg. The most commonly used medication is **methotrexate**, a drug that interferes with cell growth and can dissolve the ectopic pregnancy. Methotrexate is typically used when the ectopic pregnancy has not yet ruptured, and the woman is in stable condition. This non-invasive treatment avoids the need for surgery and can be effective if the pregnancy is detected early.

2. Surgical Treatment: If the ectopic pregnancy has progressed to a point where there is significant risk of rupture or if the woman is experiencing severe symptoms, surgery may be necessary. There are two main types of surgery:

- **Laparoscopic Surgery:** This minimally invasive surgery involves making small incisions in the abdomen and using a camera to locate and remove the ectopic pregnancy. The goal of laparoscopic surgery is to preserve as much of the fallopian tube as possible, thereby minimizing the risk of infertility.

- **Laparotomy:** In cases of severe internal bleeding or a ruptured fallopian tube, a more invasive procedure called laparotomy may be performed. This involves a larger incision to remove the ectopic pregnancy and repair any damage to the reproductive organs.

3. Expectant Management: In rare cases, when the ectopic pregnancy is very small and the woman is stable, healthcare providers may opt for expectant management. This approach involves closely monitoring the pregnancy with regular blood tests and ultrasounds to see if the body will naturally resolve the ectopic pregnancy without intervention. Expectant management is only appropriate in specific circumstances and is not commonly used.

Potential Complications

If left untreated, an ectopic pregnancy can lead to serious complications:

1. **Rupture of the Fallopian Tube:** The most dangerous complication of an ectopic pregnancy is the rupture of the fallopian tube. When the embryo grows too large for the tube, it can cause the tube to tear, leading to internal bleeding. This can be life-threatening and requires emergency surgery to stop the bleeding and repair the damage.

2. **Infertility:** Damage to the fallopian tubes from an ectopic pregnancy, particularly if surgery is required, can increase the risk of infertility. Scar tissue or adhesions may block the tubes, preventing future pregnancies from occurring. However, many women are able to conceive again after treatment for an ectopic pregnancy.

3. **Hemorrhagic Shock:** In severe cases, extensive blood loss from a ruptured ectopic pregnancy can lead to hemorrhagic shock, a condition in which the body is unable to circulate enough blood to vital organs. This requires immediate medical intervention and can be fatal if not treated promptly.

4. **Emotional Impact:** An ectopic pregnancy can also have a significant emotional toll on the woman, especially if it results in the loss of a pregnancy or affects fertility. Support from healthcare providers, mental health professionals, and support groups is essential in helping women cope with the emotional aspects of an ectopic pregnancy.

Conclusion

Ectopic pregnancy is a serious medical condition that requires prompt diagnosis and treatment to prevent complications. Although the causes and risk factors for ectopic pregnancy are varied, early detection and medical intervention can significantly reduce the risks of permanent damage and preserve the health of the woman. By understanding the symptoms, diagnostic processes, and available treatment options, women can be better equipped to recognize this condition and seek timely medical care.

Chapter 3

Ovarian Cysts: Types, Symptoms, and Treatments

Ovarian cysts are fluid-filled sacs that form within or on the surface of an ovary. They are relatively common and often occur as part of the normal functioning of the reproductive system. In most cases, ovarian cysts are benign (non-cancerous) and resolve on their own without causing significant issues. However, certain types of cysts may lead to complications, such as pain, hormonal imbalances, or difficulties with fertility. Understanding the types of ovarian cysts, their symptoms, how they affect fertility, and the treatment options available is crucial for managing these conditions effectively.

The ovaries are a pair of small, almond-shaped organs located on either side of the uterus. They are responsible for producing eggs (ova) and releasing hormones such as estrogen and progesterone, which regulate the menstrual cycle and support pregnancy. Ovarian cysts can form during the menstrual cycle, and many women will develop cysts at some point in their lives. While most ovarian cysts are harmless, others may lead to complications that require medical attention.

The Different Types of Ovarian Cysts

There are several types of ovarian cysts, each with distinct characteristics. Some cysts are functional, meaning they result from the normal process of ovulation, while others may be caused by underlying medical conditions. Below are the most common types of ovarian cysts:

1. Functional Cysts: Functional cysts are the most common type of ovarian cyst, and they typically form during the menstrual cycle. These cysts are usually benign and do not pose a serious threat to health. Functional cysts can be classified into two main types:

- **Follicular Cysts:** During the menstrual cycle, an egg is released from the follicle (the sac that holds the egg) in the process of ovulation. In some cases, the follicle does not release the egg and instead continues to grow, forming a cyst. This is known as a follicular cyst. These cysts are usually small and may resolve on their own within a few weeks.
- **Corpus Luteum Cysts:** After ovulation, the follicle transforms into the corpus luteum, a structure that produces the hormone progesterone to support a potential pregnancy. If the corpus luteum does not shrink as it should, it can fill with fluid and form a corpus luteum cyst. These cysts can cause mild pain or discomfort but are often harmless and tend to resolve naturally.

2. Dermoid Cysts (Teratomas): Dermoid cysts are less common but are made up of a variety of tissues, such as hair, skin, and fat. These cysts are usually present from birth and are classified as benign tumors. Although they are non-cancerous, dermoid cysts can grow large and cause symptoms, including pain or pressure in the pelvic area. Surgical removal may be necessary if the cyst causes significant problems.

3. Endometriomas: Endometriomas are ovarian cysts that form as a result of endometriosis, a condition in which the tissue that normally lines the inside of the uterus grows outside of it. When this tissue attaches to the ovaries, it can form cysts filled with blood. Endometriomas are often referred to as "chocolate cysts" because of the dark, thick blood inside. These cysts can cause pain, irregular periods, and can contribute to infertility. Endometriosis-related cysts often require treatment to manage symptoms and improve fertility outcomes.

4. Cystadenomas: Cystadenomas are benign ovarian cysts that develop from the cells on the outer surface of the ovary. These cysts can grow quite large and contain a watery or mucous-filled fluid. While most cystadenomas are non-cancerous, they can cause symptoms such as bloating, pelvic pressure, and pain. In rare cases, cystadenomas may become malignant, so regular monitoring or surgical removal may be necessary.

5. Polycystic Ovary Syndrome (PCOS): Polycystic ovary syndrome (PCOS) is a hormonal disorder that can cause multiple small cysts to form on the ovaries. These cysts are not true ovarian cysts but are instead underdeveloped follicles that failed to release an egg during the menstrual cycle. PCOS is associated with hormonal imbalances, including elevated levels of androgens (male hormones), which can lead to irregular periods, acne, excessive hair growth, and infertility. PCOS is a common cause of infertility and can lead to other health issues such as diabetes, obesity, and cardiovascular disease.

6. Ovarian Cancer Cysts: Although most ovarian cysts are benign, in rare cases, cysts can be cancerous. Ovarian cancer often develops silently, with few early symptoms. However, certain risk factors, such as a family history of ovarian or breast cancer, may increase the likelihood of malignant ovarian cysts. These cysts may cause more severe symptoms such as bloating, unintentional weight loss, pelvic pain, and changes in bowel habits. Early detection through screenings and diagnostic imaging is essential for improving the prognosis of ovarian cancer.

How Cysts Affect Fertility and Health

In most cases, ovarian cysts do not affect fertility, especially when they are functional cysts that resolve on their own. However, certain types of cysts and underlying conditions associated with cysts can impact fertility, menstrual cycles, and overall reproductive health.

1. Functional Cysts and Fertility: Functional cysts, such as follicular and corpus luteum cysts, are usually not associated with long-term fertility issues. These cysts tend to resolve on their own within a few weeks to months without treatment. However, recurrent functional cysts can interfere with ovulation, which may make it more difficult for a woman to conceive. If cysts persist and cause significant disruption to the menstrual cycle or hormone production, it may be necessary to seek medical intervention to manage the condition.

2. Endometriomas and Fertility: Endometriomas, often associated with endometriosis, can significantly impact fertility. Endometriosis causes the formation of scar tissue (adhesions) and cysts in the pelvic area, which can block the fallopian tubes or disrupt the ovaries' ability to release eggs. Endometriomas may also reduce the ovarian reserve, making it more difficult for women with endometriosis to conceive. Treatment for endometriomas often involves medications to manage symptoms, hormone therapy, or surgery to remove the cysts and any associated scar tissue. In severe cases, assisted reproductive technologies, such as in vitro fertilization (IVF), may be required to achieve pregnancy.

3. PCOS and Fertility: Polycystic ovary syndrome (PCOS) is a leading cause of infertility in women due to its effects on ovulation. Women with PCOS may have infrequent or absent ovulation, which prevents the release of eggs for fertilization. The cysts in PCOS are underdeveloped follicles that do not release eggs as they should. In addition to infertility, PCOS can cause hormonal imbalances that lead to irregular periods, weight gain, and symptoms such as excessive hair growth or acne. However, with proper management, such as lifestyle changes, medications to regulate ovulation, and fertility treatments like clomiphene citrate or IVF, many women with PCOS can successfully conceive.

4. Cystadenomas and Fertility: Cystadenomas are typically benign, but if they grow large or cause significant pain or discomfort, they may need to be surgically removed. Removal of cystadenomas is generally not associated with fertility issues, as long as the surgery does not damage the ovaries. However, if a cystadenoma is found to be cancerous, the treatment may involve the removal of the ovary, which can impact fertility.

5. Ovarian Cancer and Fertility: Ovarian cancer is a rare but serious cause of ovarian cysts. If detected early, ovarian cancer can be treated effectively, but advanced stages of ovarian cancer may require the removal of both ovaries, leading to infertility. Women diagnosed with ovarian cancer who wish to preserve fertility may opt for fertility preservation techniques, such as egg freezing or embryo freezing, before undergoing surgery or chemotherapy. Early diagnosis and prompt treatment are crucial for maintaining both reproductive and overall health.

Available Treatments and When Surgery is Necessary

The treatment for ovarian cysts depends on several factors, including the type of cyst, its size, whether it causes symptoms, and whether it affects fertility or general health. In many cases, ovarian cysts resolve on their own without requiring treatment. However, in cases where the cyst causes complications or persists, treatment options may include medication or surgery.

1. Observation and Monitoring: For most small, functional cysts that cause no symptoms, healthcare providers may recommend a "watch and wait" approach. This involves monitoring the cyst with periodic ultrasounds and blood tests to ensure that it resolves on its own. Functional cysts generally do not require medical treatment, as they often shrink or disappear within a few months.

2. Hormonal Birth Control: For women who experience recurrent functional cysts, hormonal birth control (such as the pill, patch, or intrauterine device) may be prescribed. Hormonal contraception can help regulate the menstrual cycle, reduce the formation of new cysts, and prevent ovulation. This treatment is often used as a preventive measure for those with frequent cyst formation.

3. Medications for Endometriomas and PCOS: For women with endometriomas or PCOS, medications may be prescribed to manage symptoms and reduce cyst formation. Hormonal therapies, such as birth control pills, progesterone, or GnRH agonists, can help regulate hormone levels, reduce cyst growth, and manage symptoms such as pain or irregular periods. In some cases, medications to induce ovulation may be used for women with PCOS who wish to conceive.

4. Surgical Treatment: Surgery is often necessary when ovarian cysts are large, painful, or do not resolve on their own. The type of surgery depends on the cyst's size, type, and whether it is benign or malignant. The two primary surgical options are:

- **Laparoscopy:** This minimally invasive surgery involves making small incisions in the abdomen and using a camera to remove the cyst. Laparoscopy is typically used for small cysts or when the cyst is non-cancerous. The goal is to remove the cyst while preserving the ovary and maintaining fertility.

- **Laparotomy:** For larger cysts or cysts that may be cancerous, a laparotomy may be necessary. This procedure involves a larger incision to access the ovary and remove the cyst. In cases of ovarian cancer, the affected ovary may be removed, which can affect fertility.

5. **Fertility Treatments:** For women with fertility issues related to ovarian cysts, fertility treatments such as ovulation induction, intrauterine insemination (IUI), or IVF may be recommended. These treatments can help women conceive even if cysts have affected their fertility.

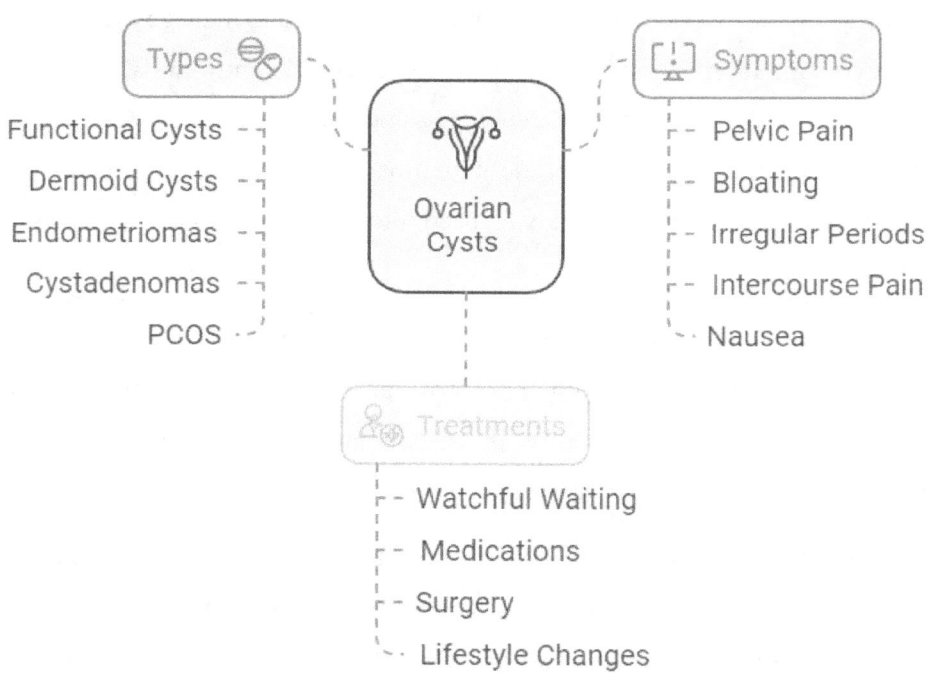

Conclusion

Ovarian cysts are common and often harmless, but some can cause significant health issues or affect fertility. The type of cyst, its size, and associated symptoms play a crucial role in determining the appropriate treatment. In many cases, ovarian cysts resolve on their own, but in other instances, medication or surgery may be necessary. For women experiencing fertility challenges, there are options available to manage cysts and improve the chances of conception. By understanding the types, symptoms, and treatments of ovarian cysts, women can make informed decisions about their health and reproductive future.

Chapter 4

Pelvic Organ Prolapse: What Every Woman Needs to Know

Introduction to Pelvic Organ Prolapse

Pelvic Organ Prolapse (POP) is a common but often under-discussed condition that affects women, particularly as they age or experience significant life changes such as childbirth or menopause. It occurs when the pelvic organs—such as the bladder, uterus, small intestine, or rectum—descend or protrude into the vaginal canal due to weakened or damaged pelvic floor muscles and connective tissues. Though pelvic organ prolapse is not always a cause for alarm, it can lead to discomfort and other health complications, significantly affecting a woman's quality of life.

Understanding the causes, symptoms, diagnosis, and treatment options for pelvic organ prolapse is crucial for women experiencing this condition. By addressing the condition early and exploring lifestyle changes or medical interventions, women can manage the symptoms and improve their overall well-being. In this chapter, we will delve into the development of POP, its clinical signs, diagnostic approaches, treatment options, and the necessary lifestyle modifications that can alleviate symptoms and promote long-term pelvic health.

How Pelvic Organ Prolapse Develops

Pelvic organ prolapse develops as a result of the weakening or stretching of the pelvic floor muscles and ligaments that support the pelvic organs. The pelvic floor is a group of muscles and tissues located at the bottom of the pelvis. These muscles form a "hammock" that supports the bladder, uterus, vagina, rectum, and small intestines. When these muscles become weakened, damaged, or overstretched, they lose their ability to hold the pelvic organs in place, leading to prolapse.

Several factors contribute to the development of pelvic organ prolapse, including:

1. **Childbirth:** One of the most common causes of pelvic organ prolapse is vaginal childbirth, particularly when the delivery is complicated or involves prolonged labor, the use of forceps, or delivery of a large baby. The strain of pregnancy and childbirth can cause the pelvic floor muscles to stretch or tear, making them less effective at supporting the organs. Multiple vaginal deliveries increase the risk of prolapse, especially in older women or those with large babies.

2. **Aging and Menopause:** As women age, the body undergoes hormonal changes, especially the decline in estrogen levels that occurs after menopause. Estrogen plays a key role in maintaining the strength and integrity of the pelvic tissues. Without sufficient estrogen, the pelvic muscles and connective tissues weaken, increasing the risk of prolapse. Older women, particularly those who have had multiple children or have experienced the natural process of aging, are at a higher risk.

3. **Chronic Pressure on the Pelvic Floor:** Chronic conditions that increase pressure on the pelvic floor can contribute to prolapse. These conditions include chronic constipation, obesity, heavy lifting, chronic coughing (such as in smokers or those with respiratory conditions), and frequent straining during bowel movements. Increased pressure can weaken the pelvic floor over time, leading to prolapse.

4. **Genetics:** Genetics can play a role in the development of pelvic organ prolapse. Some women may have a hereditary predisposition to weak pelvic floor muscles and connective tissues, making them more susceptible to prolapse. If a woman has a family history of POP, she may be at a higher risk.

5. **Previous Pelvic Surgery:** Women who have had previous pelvic surgeries, such as a hysterectomy (removal of the uterus), may be at increased risk of developing pelvic organ prolapse. Surgery can weaken the pelvic floor muscles or disrupt the supportive structures, leading to a higher likelihood of prolapse in the future.

6. **Other Factors:** Other conditions, such as neurological disorders or connective tissue disorders like Ehlers-Danlos syndrome, may increase the likelihood of prolapse. Women who have experienced significant trauma to the pelvic area or who have chronic pelvic infections may also be more vulnerable to prolapse.

Symptoms of Pelvic Organ Prolapse

The symptoms of pelvic organ prolapse can vary depending on the severity of the condition and the specific pelvic organ involved. Many women with prolapse experience only mild symptoms or may not experience any symptoms at all. However, in more severe cases, prolapse can significantly affect a woman's physical, emotional, and social well-being. Common symptoms of pelvic organ prolapse include:

1. **A Feeling of Fullness or Pressure in the Pelvis:** Women with pelvic organ prolapse may experience a sensation of heaviness, fullness, or pressure in the pelvic area. This feeling may worsen as the day progresses or with activities

such as standing, walking, or lifting. The sensation may feel as though something is "falling out" of the vagina.

2. **Protrusion or Bulging in the Vaginal Area:** In more advanced cases of prolapse, women may notice a visible bulge or protrusion from the vaginal opening. This bulge is often more prominent when standing or during activities that put pressure on the pelvic floor, such as coughing or straining.

3. **Urinary Symptoms:** Pelvic organ prolapse can interfere with normal urinary function. Women may experience urinary incontinence (leakage of urine), a frequent need to urinate, difficulty emptying the bladder completely, or urinary retention. In severe cases, prolapse can lead to a urinary tract infection (UTI) due to incomplete bladder emptying.

4. **Bowel Problems:** Prolapse can also affect bowel function. Women with pelvic organ prolapse may have difficulty with bowel movements, experience constipation, or feel the need to strain excessively. In some cases, prolapse can cause rectal prolapse (when part of the rectum protrudes through the anus), leading to a feeling of incomplete evacuation or difficulty controlling bowel movements.

5. **Pain or Discomfort:** While many women with prolapse do not experience significant pain, some may feel pelvic pain, lower back pain, or discomfort during sexual intercourse. In more advanced cases, prolapse can lead to pain in the pelvic region due to the excessive pressure on the organs and surrounding muscles.

6. **Sexual Dysfunction:** Women with pelvic organ prolapse may experience discomfort or pain during sexual intercourse due to the protrusion of pelvic organs into the vaginal canal. In some cases, prolapse can make sexual

activity difficult or unenjoyable, leading to a reduction in sexual desire and intimacy issues.

Diagnosis of Pelvic Organ Prolapse

The diagnosis of pelvic organ prolapse begins with a thorough medical history and physical examination. During the examination, a healthcare provider may ask about symptoms, lifestyle habits, and any relevant medical history, such as previous pregnancies, surgeries, or pelvic conditions.

The provider will typically perform a pelvic exam to evaluate the degree of prolapse and determine which pelvic organs are involved. During this exam, the patient may be asked to cough or bear down to increase pressure on the pelvic floor and help the provider identify any organ descent. In some cases, a woman may also undergo additional tests to assess the function of the bladder and bowel, such as urodynamic testing or imaging studies.

If prolapse is suspected, imaging techniques such as ultrasound or MRI may be used to evaluate the extent of the prolapse and rule out other potential causes of symptoms.

Treatment Options for Pelvic Organ Prolapse

The treatment for pelvic organ prolapse depends on the severity of the condition, the symptoms experienced, and the woman's overall health and preferences. Treatment can be categorized into non-surgical (conservative) and surgical options.

1. Non-Surgical Treatment Options:

- **Pelvic Floor Exercises (Kegel Exercises):** Kegel exercises, which involve tightening and relaxing the pelvic floor muscles, can strengthen the muscles supporting the pelvic organs. Regular practice of Kegels can improve symptoms of prolapse, reduce pressure in the pelvic area, and help prevent the condition from worsening.

- **Pessaries:** A pessary is a device that is inserted into the vagina to support the prolapsed organs. It is often used for women who are not ready for surgery or are not good candidates for surgical interventions. Pessaries come in different shapes and sizes, and a healthcare provider will help determine the best fit for each woman. Pessaries can provide significant relief of symptoms, particularly the feeling of bulging or pressure in the pelvis.

- **Lifestyle Modifications:** Certain lifestyle changes can help reduce the symptoms of prolapse and prevent the condition from worsening. These include maintaining a healthy weight, avoiding heavy lifting, managing constipation, and practicing good posture. Regular physical activity, including exercises to strengthen the core and pelvic muscles, can also be beneficial.

- **Hormonal Therapy:** For women experiencing pelvic organ prolapse due to menopause or hormonal changes, estrogen therapy may be recommended to improve the strength and elasticity of pelvic tissues. Estrogen can be applied locally in the form of creams, rings, or tablets to target the pelvic area without affecting the rest of the body.

2. Surgical Treatment Options:

When conservative treatments are ineffective or when prolapse is severe, surgery may be necessary to correct the condition. Surgical options include:

- **Anterior or Posterior Repair:** In cases where the bladder or rectum is prolapsed, surgery can be performed to repair the walls of the vagina and reposition the organs. Anterior repair addresses the front vaginal wall (bladder prolapse), while posterior repair addresses the back wall (rectal prolapse).

- **Vaginal Hysterectomy:** For women with uterine prolapse, a vaginal hysterectomy may be performed to remove the uterus. This surgery may be done in conjunction with repairs to other prolapsed organs.

- **Sacrocolpopexy:** This surgery involves attaching the vaginal vault (post-hysterectomy) or the cervix to the sacrum (a bone at the base of the spine) to support the prolapsed organs. It is typically performed through a minimally invasive laparoscopic approach.

- **Colpocleisis:** Colpocleisis is a surgical procedure used for women who are not sexually active or no longer wish to preserve vaginal function. It involves closing off the vaginal canal to prevent further prolapse of the pelvic organs.

Lifestyle Changes for Managing Pelvic Organ Prolapse

In addition to medical treatments, certain lifestyle changes can help women manage pelvic organ prolapse and reduce symptoms:

1. **Maintain a Healthy Weight:** Excess weight places additional pressure on the pelvic floor muscles, exacerbating prolapse symptoms. Maintaining a healthy weight through diet and exercise can reduce strain on the pelvic region.

2. **Avoid Heavy Lifting:** Lifting heavy objects puts significant pressure on the pelvic floor. If heavy lifting is unavoidable, it's essential to use proper lifting techniques and engage the pelvic floor muscles to help support the organs.

3. **Treat Constipation:** Chronic constipation can worsen pelvic organ prolapse by increasing strain during bowel movements. Eating a fiber-rich diet, staying hydrated, and incorporating regular exercise can promote healthy bowel function and reduce constipation.

4. **Practice Good Posture:** Maintaining good posture can help reduce pressure on the pelvic floor muscles. Standing and sitting with proper alignment can alleviate strain on the pelvic region and help manage symptoms.

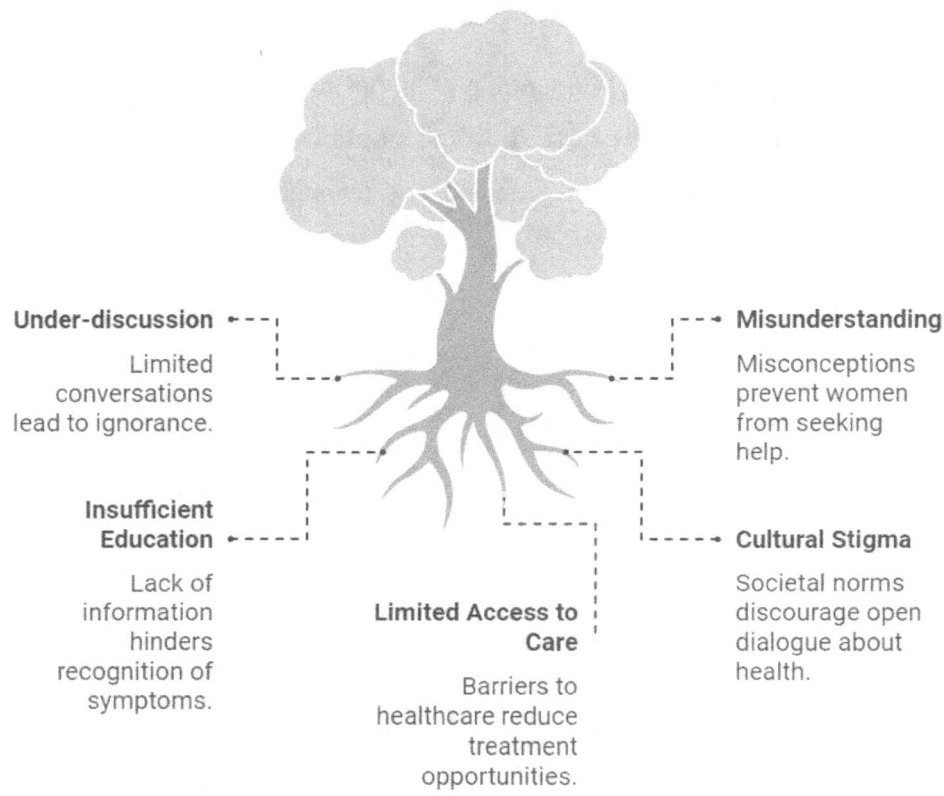

Lack of Awareness about Pelvic Organ Prolapse

Under-discussion
Limited conversations lead to ignorance.

Misunderstanding
Misconceptions prevent women from seeking help.

Insufficient Education
Lack of information hinders recognition of symptoms.

Limited Access to Care
Barriers to healthcare reduce treatment opportunities.

Cultural Stigma
Societal norms discourage open dialogue about health.

Conclusion

Pelvic organ prolapse is a condition that affects many women, especially as they age or experience life changes such as childbirth or menopause. While prolapse can be distressing, it is a treatable condition with various management options. By understanding the causes, recognizing the symptoms, and exploring both non-surgical and surgical treatment options, women can take control of their pelvic health and improve their quality of life. Early diagnosis, lifestyle modifications, and personalized medical care are key to successfully managing pelvic organ prolapse and promoting long-term pelvic health.

Chapter 5

Uterine Fibroids: Causes, Symptoms, and Management

Introduction to Uterine Fibroids

Uterine fibroids, also known as myomas or leiomyomas, are non-cancerous tumors that develop in the muscle tissue of the uterus. These growths are incredibly common, with studies indicating that up to 70-80% of women will have fibroids by the time they reach 50 years of age. While many women with uterine fibroids experience no symptoms, for others, the condition can lead to significant discomfort and health complications, especially in terms of fertility, menstrual health, and quality of life.

Fibroids vary in size, shape, and location within the uterus. Some may be as small as a pea, while others can grow large enough to distort the shape of the uterus. They can be found on the outer surface of the uterus (subserosal fibroids), within the muscle of the uterus (intramural fibroids), or inside the uterine cavity (submucosal fibroids). Understanding what uterine fibroids are, their causes, symptoms, and available treatment options is critical for managing the condition and improving a woman's overall health.

What Uterine Fibroids Are and Why They Form

Uterine fibroids are benign tumors made up of smooth muscle and fibrous tissue. They develop in the uterus, typically during the reproductive years, and can vary greatly in size. Although fibroids are non-cancerous, their growth can lead to a variety of symptoms depending on their size, number, and location. Most fibroids grow slowly, and in many cases, they do not cause any symptoms at all. However, in some women, they can lead to problems that affect daily life.

The exact cause of uterine fibroids remains unclear, but there are several factors believed to contribute to their development:

1. **Hormonal Influence:** Estrogen and progesterone, two hormones that regulate the female reproductive system, are believed to stimulate the growth of fibroids. These hormones promote the growth of smooth muscle cells in the uterus, and higher levels of estrogen are thought to be particularly influential. This is one of the reasons why fibroids are more common in women of reproductive age and tend to shrink after menopause when estrogen levels decrease.

2. **Genetic Factors:** There is evidence to suggest that genetics play a role in the development of uterine fibroids. Women with a family history of fibroids are more likely to develop them themselves. Certain genetic mutations have been associated with fibroid growth, and researchers continue to investigate how these genetic factors influence fibroid formation.

3. **Cellular Changes:** Fibroids arise from the smooth muscle cells in the uterus, which undergo abnormal growth. While normal uterine muscle cells grow and divide in a controlled manner, the cells that form fibroids exhibit uncontrolled growth, leading to the formation of tumors. Some studies suggest that fibroids may result from a response to injury or inflammation within the uterus, although this hypothesis requires more research.

4. **Lifestyle and Environmental Factors:** Although less well-established, certain lifestyle factors may contribute to fibroid development. Obesity, for instance, has been associated with an increased risk of developing fibroids, possibly due to higher levels of estrogen produced in fatty tissue. High blood

pressure and diet, particularly a diet high in red meat and low in fruits and vegetables, may also contribute to the risk of fibroid formation.

5. **Age and Ethnicity:** Uterine fibroids are most common in women between the ages of 30 and 50, with the risk decreasing after menopause. African American women are at higher risk of developing fibroids compared to women of other ethnic backgrounds, and they may also experience more severe symptoms and larger fibroids. Race and ethnicity are thought to influence the size, number, and severity of fibroids, though the reasons for these disparities are still being researched.

Symptom Severity and When to Seek Treatment

The majority of women with uterine fibroids experience no symptoms, and many may be unaware of their condition until they undergo a routine pelvic exam or ultrasound. However, when symptoms do occur, they can range from mild to severe, and the impact on a woman's life can be significant.

Common symptoms of uterine fibroids include:

1. **Heavy Menstrual Bleeding:** One of the most common symptoms of uterine fibroids is abnormal or heavy menstrual bleeding, often described as flooding or prolonged periods. This can lead to anemia (low iron levels) and fatigue, and may require frequent changes in sanitary products during menstruation.

2. **Pelvic Pain and Pressure:** Fibroids can cause pelvic pain or a feeling of fullness or pressure in the lower abdomen. Large fibroids can press on nearby organs, such as the bladder or rectum, leading to discomfort or a sensation of heaviness. Some women also report pain during sexual intercourse.

3. **Frequent Urination:** If fibroids grow near the bladder, they can cause frequent urination or difficulty emptying the bladder completely. This occurs due to pressure on the bladder, which reduces its capacity to hold urine.

4. **Constipation:** When fibroids press on the rectum, they can cause constipation, difficulty with bowel movements, or a sensation of incomplete evacuation. Some women may experience bloating or swelling in the lower abdomen as well.

5. **Infertility and Pregnancy Complications:** In some cases, uterine fibroids can interfere with fertility. Large or multiple fibroids may block the fallopian tubes, impair embryo implantation, or alter the shape of the uterine cavity, making it difficult for a woman to conceive. Fibroids may also increase the risk of complications during pregnancy, including miscarriage, preterm labor, or a breech presentation.

6. **Back or Leg Pain:** Large fibroids can cause pain in the lower back or legs due to their size and pressure on surrounding tissues. This can affect a woman's mobility and comfort during daily activities.

7. **Enlarged Abdomen:** In rare cases, particularly with very large fibroids, women may notice a visible enlargement of the abdomen, resembling pregnancy. This is typically associated with significant fibroid growth and may cause a bloated or distended appearance.

If you experience any of the symptoms listed above, particularly heavy bleeding, pelvic pain, or difficulty with urination or bowel movements, it is essential to seek medical attention. In addition, if fibroids are interfering with fertility or causing pregnancy complications, timely treatment is necessary to preserve reproductive health. A healthcare provider can evaluate the severity of your symptoms and recommend appropriate treatment options based on your individual circumstances.

Non-Surgical Treatment Options for Uterine Fibroids

For many women, non-surgical treatment options can help manage the symptoms of uterine fibroids without the need for invasive procedures. These options are typically suitable for women with smaller fibroids or those who do not wish to undergo surgery for personal, health, or fertility reasons. Non-surgical treatments aim to alleviate symptoms, reduce fibroid size, or improve quality of life.

1. **Medications:** Several medications are used to manage fibroid symptoms, particularly heavy bleeding and pain:

    - **Hormonal Treatments:** Birth control pills, hormonal IUDs, or hormone therapy can help regulate menstrual cycles and reduce bleeding. The hormonal IUD, in particular, can help with heavy periods by thinning the uterine lining and decreasing bleeding.

    - **GnRH Agonists:** Gonadotropin-releasing hormone (GnRH) agonists are medications that temporarily shrink fibroids by lowering estrogen levels. These drugs put women into a temporary menopause-like state, which reduces the size of fibroids and alleviates symptoms. However, GnRH agonists are typically used for short periods due to their side effects, such as hot flashes and bone density loss.

    - **Tranexamic Acid:** This medication can be used to reduce heavy menstrual bleeding by promoting blood clotting. It is often prescribed for women with fibroids who experience excessive bleeding during their periods.

2. **Uterine Artery Embolization (UAE):** UAE is a minimally invasive procedure used to shrink fibroids by blocking the blood supply that nourishes them. A catheter is inserted into the uterine artery through a small incision in the groin, and small particles are injected to block the blood vessels feeding the fibroids. This causes the fibroids to shrink and symptoms to improve. UAE is an effective treatment option for women who do not want to undergo surgery and have no desire for future pregnancies.

3. **MRI-Guided Focused Ultrasound (MRgFUS):** This is a non-invasive treatment that uses focused ultrasound waves, guided by MRI imaging, to target and destroy fibroid tissue. The procedure is typically used for women with smaller fibroids who are experiencing significant symptoms. It is considered a safe and effective alternative to traditional surgery, although it may not be suitable for all women.

4. **Lifestyle Changes:** In addition to medical treatments, certain lifestyle changes may help alleviate fibroid symptoms. Maintaining a healthy weight, eating a balanced diet, and engaging in regular exercise may help reduce the size of fibroids or prevent their growth. Managing stress and avoiding substances that increase estrogen levels, such as excessive alcohol or smoking, can also be beneficial.

Surgical Treatment Options for Uterine Fibroids

For women with large, multiple, or symptomatic fibroids that do not respond to non-surgical treatments, surgery may be necessary. The goal of surgery is to remove or shrink fibroids, restore normal uterine function, and relieve symptoms. Several surgical options are available, depending on the severity of the condition and the woman's reproductive goals.

1. **Myomectomy:** A myomectomy is a surgical procedure in which fibroids are removed from the uterus. This option is often recommended for women who wish to preserve their fertility. The fibroids are carefully excised, and the uterus is sutured back together. Myomectomy can be performed via different techniques, including abdominal, laparoscopic, or hysteroscopic surgery, depending on the size, location, and number of fibroids.

2. **Hysterectomy:** For women who no longer wish to have children or who have severe fibroids that do not respond to other treatments, a hysterectomy may be recommended. This procedure involves the complete removal of the uterus and, in some cases, the removal of the ovaries and fallopian tubes as well. A hysterectomy offers a permanent solution to fibroids and eliminates the possibility of future fibroid development.

3. **Endometrial Ablation:** Endometrial ablation is a procedure used to destroy the lining of the uterus, which can help control heavy bleeding caused by fibroids. While this procedure is effective at reducing bleeding, it is not suitable for women who wish to preserve fertility, as it may interfere with implantation or pregnancy.

4. **Laparoscopic or Robotic Surgery:** In some cases, fibroids can be removed using minimally invasive techniques, such as laparoscopic or robotic-assisted surgery. These approaches involve smaller incisions and a quicker recovery time compared to traditional open surgery.

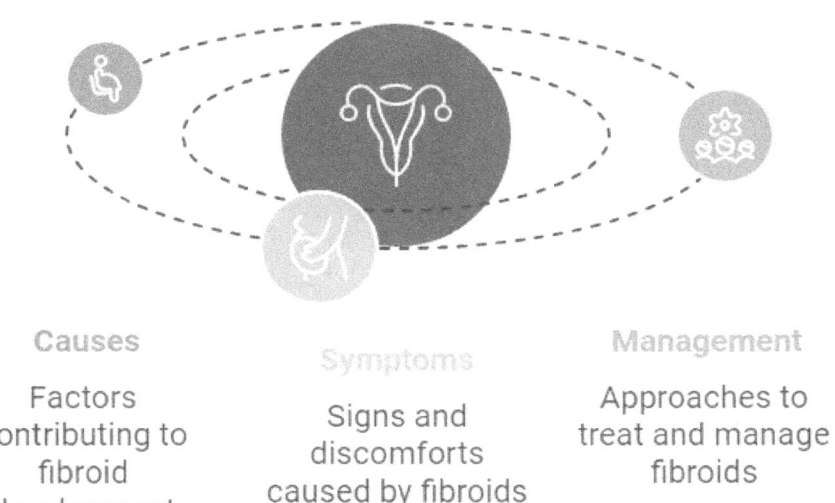

Understanding Uterine Fibroids

Causes — Factors contributing to fibroid development

Symptoms — Signs and discomforts caused by fibroids

Management — Approaches to treat and manage fibroids

Conclusion

Uterine fibroids are common and, in many cases, non-cancerous tumors that cause a variety of symptoms for women. While many women live with fibroids without significant problems, others experience debilitating symptoms that require medical intervention. By understanding the causes of fibroids, recognizing the signs and symptoms, and exploring treatment options, women can make informed decisions about their health. Whether opting for non-surgical treatments like medication or procedures such as UAE and MRgFUS, or pursuing surgery, such as myomectomy or hysterectomy, women can manage their fibroid symptoms and lead healthier, more comfortable lives. It is essential to work closely with a healthcare provider to determine the best treatment plan based on individual needs, reproductive goals, and overall health.

Chapter 6

Endometrial Cancer: Early Detection and Treatment

Understanding Endometrial Cancer and Risk Factors

Endometrial cancer, also known as uterine cancer, is the most common cancer of the female reproductive system. It originates in the lining of the uterus, called the endometrium, which thickens and sheds during the menstrual cycle. When the cells of the endometrium begin to grow abnormally and uncontrollably, they can form a tumor. If left untreated, these cancerous cells can spread to other parts of the body.

The majority of endometrial cancers are classified as *endometrioid adenocarcinomas*, which are associated with abnormal hormone levels, particularly estrogen. This type of cancer tends to develop slowly, often giving women the opportunity to catch it in its early stages, when treatment is most effective.

Understanding the risk factors for endometrial cancer is crucial for early detection and prevention. While any woman can develop endometrial cancer, certain factors can increase the likelihood of its occurrence. These factors include:

1. **Age:**
   The risk of endometrial cancer increases with age, particularly after menopause. Most cases are diagnosed in women over 50, with the average age of diagnosis being 60. Postmenopausal women with unusual vaginal bleeding should be promptly evaluated for possible endometrial cancer.

2. **Hormonal Imbalances:**
   An excess of estrogen without the balancing effect of progesterone is a key risk factor. Conditions such as polycystic ovary syndrome (PCOS), obesity,

or hormone replacement therapy (HRT) can lead to an imbalance, which may increase the risk of endometrial cancer. Women who have never been pregnant or who experience prolonged exposure to estrogen without progesterone are also at higher risk.

3. **Obesity:**

   Women with a higher body mass index (BMI) are at increased risk due to the role fat cells play in producing estrogen. Excess fat, especially abdominal fat, can lead to higher estrogen levels in the body, increasing the risk of developing endometrial cancer.

4. **Reproductive History:**

   Women who have never been pregnant or who have a history of infertility may be at higher risk of developing endometrial cancer. Additionally, women who have irregular menstrual cycles or have experienced early menstruation or late menopause are also at increased risk.

5. **Genetic Factors:**

   Certain inherited genetic conditions can increase the risk of developing endometrial cancer. The most notable of these is Lynch syndrome, also known as hereditary nonpolyposis colorectal cancer (HNPCC). Women with Lynch syndrome have a higher lifetime risk of developing endometrial cancer, often at a younger age.

6. **Diabetes:**

   Diabetes, particularly type 2 diabetes, is linked with a higher risk of endometrial cancer, possibly due to hormonal and metabolic changes associated with the condition.

7. **Family History:**
   A family history of endometrial cancer or other cancers, such as colorectal or ovarian cancer, can increase a woman's risk, especially if close relatives have been affected.

   Signs and Symptoms to Watch For

   One of the most important aspects of managing endometrial cancer is early detection. The earlier the cancer is found, the higher the chances of successful treatment. Unfortunately, the symptoms of endometrial cancer often resemble those of other benign gynecological conditions, which is why it is important for women to pay attention to any unusual or persistent signs.

1. **Unusual Vaginal Bleeding:**
   The most common and telling symptom of endometrial cancer is abnormal vaginal bleeding. Women who have gone through menopause and suddenly experience vaginal bleeding should seek medical attention immediately. Even those who have irregular periods before menopause should report any sudden changes in bleeding patterns, including very heavy or prolonged bleeding, or spotting between periods.

2. **Pelvic Pain or Discomfort:**
   Although pelvic pain is not an early sign, it can occur in the later stages of endometrial cancer. This pain may be dull and persistent or sharp and intermittent. It may be associated with a feeling of fullness or bloating in the abdomen.

3. **Pain During Intercourse (Dyspareunia):**
   Painful intercourse can be a sign of advanced endometrial cancer. This may occur if the tumor has spread to the surrounding tissues or the vaginal walls.

4. **Unexplained Weight Loss:**
Unexplained weight loss, especially when accompanied by other symptoms such as fatigue and abdominal discomfort, may be a sign of cancer. As the tumor grows, the body may react by burning more energy, leading to weight loss.

5. **Urinary Symptoms:**
In some cases, endometrial cancer can cause urinary problems, such as frequent urination or difficulty emptying the bladder. This may occur if the tumor grows and puts pressure on the bladder.

6. **Swelling in the Legs:**
As the cancer spreads to the pelvic area or other parts of the body, it can cause lymphatic blockages or other issues that lead to swelling, particularly in the legs. This is usually a sign of advanced cancer.

It is important to note that these symptoms are not exclusive to endometrial cancer, and they may occur with other, less serious conditions. However, if these symptoms persist, or if there are any sudden changes in bleeding patterns, it is essential to consult a healthcare provider for evaluation.

Available Treatments for Endometrial Cancer

Once endometrial cancer is diagnosed, treatment options will depend on several factors, including the stage of cancer, the woman's age, overall health, and whether she desires to retain her fertility. The most common treatments for endometrial cancer include surgery, radiation therapy, and chemotherapy.

1. **Surgery:**

- **Hysterectomy:**
    Surgery is the primary treatment for endometrial cancer and typically involves the removal of the uterus. In most cases, this is done through a total hysterectomy, which includes the removal of the uterus and cervix. If the cancer has spread to nearby tissues or organs, a more extensive surgery may be required. This can involve the removal of the ovaries, fallopian tubes, and surrounding lymph nodes (lymphadenectomy).

- **Minimally Invasive Surgery:**
    Depending on the stage and location of the cancer, surgery may be done using minimally invasive techniques, such as laparoscopic or robotic-assisted surgery. These methods involve smaller incisions, leading to a quicker recovery time and less postoperative pain.

- **Fertility-Sparing Surgery:**
    In cases where the cancer is confined to the lining of the uterus and the woman is of reproductive age, fertility-sparing surgery may be an option. This involves removing the cancerous tissue while preserving the uterus and ovaries. However, this approach is only suitable for early-stage cancer and must be carefully considered by the patient and her doctor.

2. **Radiation Therapy:**

Radiation therapy uses high-energy X-rays to target and destroy cancer cells. This treatment is often recommended after surgery to kill any remaining cancer cells that might not have been removed. Radiation can also be used to shrink tumors before surgery to make them easier to remove or to alleviate symptoms in advanced-stage cancers.

- **External Beam Radiation:**
  This method involves directing radiation beams from outside the body to the area affected by cancer. The treatment is non-invasive and typically given in multiple sessions over a period of several weeks.

- **Brachytherapy:**
  In some cases, radioactive material may be placed directly inside the uterus or near the tumor in a procedure called brachytherapy. This allows for a more concentrated dose of radiation to target the cancerous cells while minimizing damage to surrounding healthy tissue.

3. **Chemotherapy:**

Chemotherapy involves the use of drugs that kill cancer cells or prevent them from growing and dividing. This treatment is typically used for advanced stages of endometrial cancer or when the cancer has spread beyond the uterus. Chemotherapy can be administered intravenously or, in some cases, orally. It is often combined with surgery or radiation therapy to increase the chances of eradicating the cancer.

- **Adjuvant Chemotherapy:**
  This refers to chemotherapy given after surgery to destroy any remaining cancer cells and reduce the risk of recurrence.

- **Neoadjuvant Chemotherapy:**
  In some cases, chemotherapy may be used before surgery to shrink the

tumor and make it easier to remove. This approach is typically reserved for more advanced cancers.

4. **Hormone Therapy:**

Hormone therapy may be used for women with certain types of endometrial cancer that are hormone receptor-positive. This type of therapy works by blocking the hormones that fuel the growth of cancer cells, particularly estrogen. Medications such as progesterone, megestrol acetate, or tamoxifen can be used to manage hormone-sensitive endometrial cancer.

5. **Targeted Therapy and Immunotherapy:**

Newer treatments like targeted therapy and immunotherapy are also being explored for endometrial cancer. These treatments work by targeting specific molecules or proteins involved in cancer cell growth or boosting the body's immune response to cancer. While these therapies show promise, they are typically used in clinical trials or for women with advanced cancer who have not responded to traditional treatments.

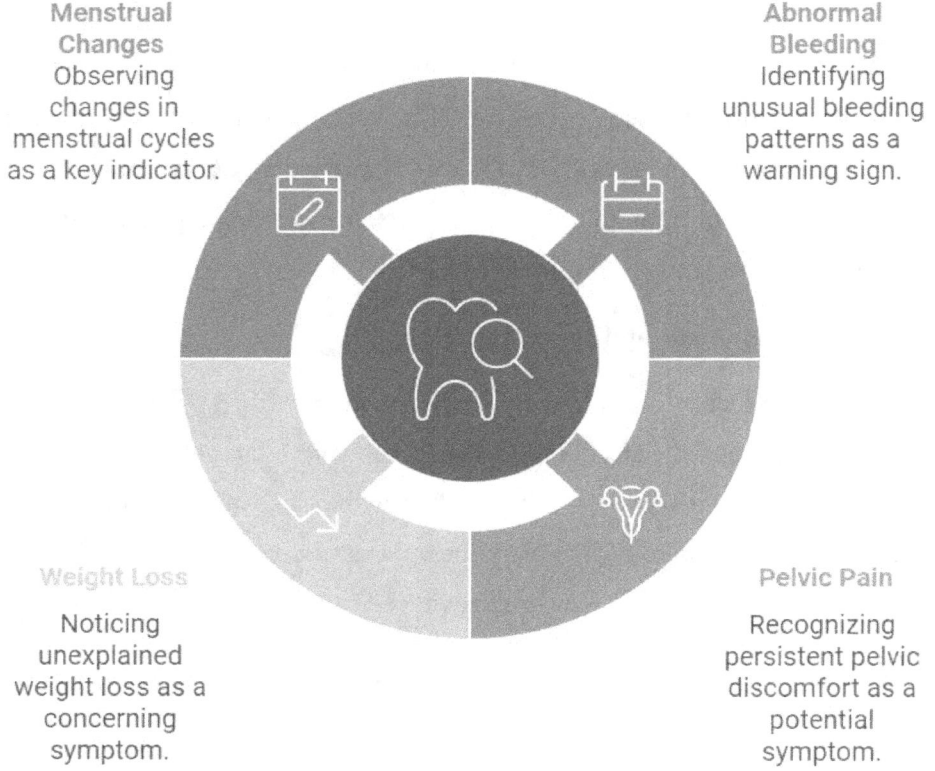

Conclusion

Endometrial cancer is a serious but treatable condition when detected early. With advances in screening, diagnosis, and treatment options, women who are at risk or experience symptoms can seek medical advice and take proactive steps for early detection. The treatment journey often involves a combination of surgery, radiation, and chemotherapy, tailored to each woman's specific situation. By understanding the risk factors, being aware of symptoms, and exploring the available treatment options, women can make informed decisions and increase their chances of successful treatment and recovery. Regular gynecological exams, monitoring for abnormal bleeding, and maintaining a healthy lifestyle are key components of reducing the risk of endometrial cancer and ensuring optimal health.

Chapter 7

Premature Ovarian Failure: The Impact on Fertility

Understanding Premature Ovarian Failure

Premature ovarian failure (POF), also known as primary ovarian insufficiency (POI), refers to the loss of normal ovarian function before the age of 40. This condition is characterized by the ovaries no longer producing eggs regularly or adequately, resulting in infertility and a range of hormonal imbalances. It is a relatively uncommon condition, affecting approximately 1 in 100 women under 40, but it can have significant consequences on a woman's fertility, hormonal health, and overall well-being.

The ovaries are responsible for producing eggs (ova) and releasing them during ovulation. In addition, they produce hormones such as estrogen and progesterone, which regulate the menstrual cycle, support pregnancy, and maintain bone health. In women with premature ovarian failure, the ovaries may stop functioning entirely or produce very few eggs, leading to a deficiency in these essential hormones.

Premature ovarian failure differs from menopause, which is a natural life stage that typically occurs between the ages of 45 and 55. In menopause, the ovaries gradually cease functioning, but this process happens over several years. In contrast, premature ovarian failure is an abrupt and premature cessation of ovarian function, often with sudden onset.

Causes of Premature Ovarian Failure

The exact cause of premature ovarian failure is not always clear, and in many cases, it occurs without any obvious reason. However, several factors and conditions are known to contribute to the development of POF.

1. **Genetic Factors**:

    Genetic mutations or abnormalities are among the most common causes of premature ovarian failure. Women with certain genetic disorders are at a higher risk of developing POF. One of the most notable is **Turner syndrome**, a genetic condition in which one of the X chromosomes is missing or incomplete. This condition often leads to ovarian dysfunction. Other genetic conditions, such as **fragile X syndrome**, can also increase the risk of early ovarian failure, especially in women who carry the fragile X mutation.

2. **Autoimmune Disorders**:

    In autoimmune conditions, the immune system mistakenly attacks the body's own tissues, and in the case of POF, the immune system may target the ovaries, leading to inflammation and damage. Women with autoimmune diseases, such as **rheumatoid arthritis**, **lupus**, or **thyroid disorders**, have a higher risk of premature ovarian failure.

3. **Chemotherapy and Radiation Therapy**:

    Cancer treatments, such as chemotherapy and radiation therapy, can significantly affect ovarian function. Both chemotherapy drugs and radiation treatments, especially those targeting the pelvic area, can damage the eggs in the ovaries, leading to premature ovarian failure. While some women may recover ovarian function after completing treatment, others may experience permanent infertility due to this damage.

4. **Surgical Removal of Ovaries**:

    In certain cases, women may undergo surgery to remove one or both ovaries due to conditions such as ovarian cysts, endometriosis, or ovarian cancer. Removal of the ovaries (oophorectomy) directly causes infertility, but it may also induce premature ovarian failure if only one ovary is removed. Furthermore, certain surgical procedures may damage ovarian blood flow, leading to decreased ovarian function.

5. **Infections**:

   Certain viral or bacterial infections can affect ovarian function. For example, infections like **mumps** or **tuberculosis** have been linked to ovarian dysfunction in some women. However, these types of infections are relatively rare causes of premature ovarian failure.

6. **Environmental Toxins**:

   Exposure to environmental toxins, such as pesticides, chemicals, and industrial pollutants, can negatively impact ovarian health. Chemicals that disrupt hormonal balance, known as endocrine disruptors, may play a role in the development of POF. Women who are exposed to high levels of such toxins may experience a higher risk of early ovarian decline.

7. **Lifestyle Factors**:

   Certain lifestyle factors, such as smoking and excessive alcohol consumption, can contribute to ovarian failure. Smoking, in particular, has been shown to decrease ovarian reserve and accelerate the onset of menopause. Women who smoke are more likely to experience POF at an earlier age compared to non-smokers.

8. **Idiopathic Causes**:

   In many cases, no clear cause for premature ovarian failure is identified. This is referred to as **idiopathic POF**, where the exact reason for ovarian dysfunction remains unknown. Genetic factors may play a role, but a definitive cause cannot always be pinpointed.

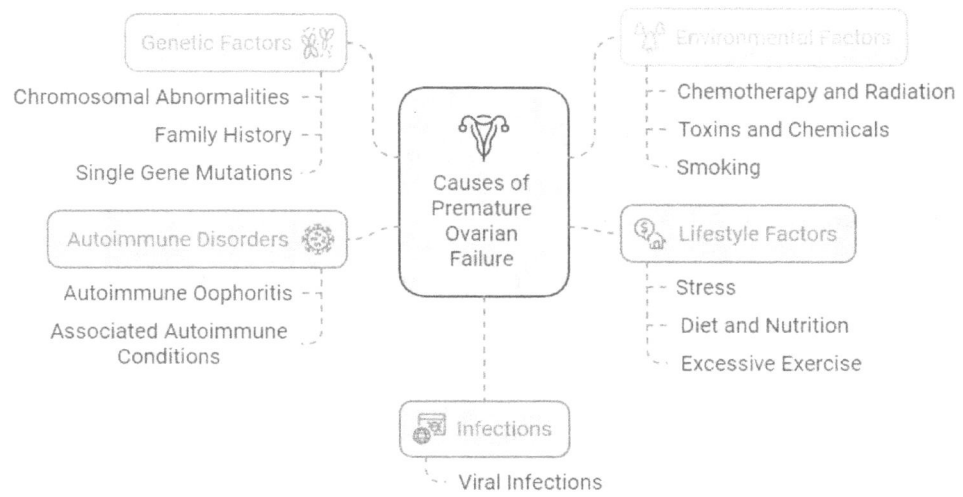

Symptoms and Diagnosis of Premature Ovarian Failure

The symptoms of premature ovarian failure can vary widely among women, and some may not experience obvious signs until they begin to struggle with infertility. The symptoms are often similar to those of menopause, although they may occur at an earlier age.

1. **Irregular or Absent Periods**:

    The most common symptom of POF is the sudden or gradual cessation of menstrual periods. Many women experience irregular periods or missed cycles before their periods completely stop. In some cases, periods may become lighter or less frequent, followed by complete cessation. Women with irregular or absent periods before the age of 40 should consult a healthcare provider for evaluation.

2. **Hot Flashes and Night Sweats**:

   As the ovaries stop producing estrogen, women with premature ovarian failure may experience symptoms typical of menopause, including hot flashes and night sweats. These can be uncomfortable and disruptive to daily life, and they may signal a decrease in ovarian function.

3. **Mood Swings and Irritability**:

   Hormonal imbalances caused by the cessation of ovarian function can lead to mood swings, irritability, and even anxiety or depression. These symptoms are often overlooked or attributed to other causes, but they are important to monitor as they can significantly affect a woman's quality of life.

4. **Decreased Libido**:

   A decrease in estrogen levels can lead to a reduced interest in sexual activity, which may be accompanied by vaginal dryness and discomfort during intercourse. These symptoms can affect relationships and emotional well-being.

5. **Infertility**:

   The most significant impact of premature ovarian failure is on fertility. Women with POF typically experience infertility because their ovaries are no longer producing eggs. This is often the first indication of POF, as many women seek medical help when they are unable to conceive despite trying for an extended period of time.

6. **Other Symptoms**:

   In addition to the above symptoms, women may also experience other signs of hormonal imbalance, such as fatigue, headaches, and difficulty concentrating. Reduced bone density (osteoporosis) may also occur due to the lack of estrogen, making bones more fragile and prone to fractures.

To diagnose premature ovarian failure, healthcare providers typically conduct a series of tests. These may include:

- **Blood Tests**:
  Blood tests to measure levels of **follicle-stimulating hormone (FSH)**, **estradiol**, and **anti-Müllerian hormone (AMH)** can help assess ovarian function. Elevated FSH levels and low estradiol levels are typically indicative of ovarian failure. AMH is often used as a marker of ovarian reserve, and low levels can suggest a diminished egg supply.

- **Ultrasound**:
  Pelvic ultrasound may be performed to assess the ovaries' size and appearance, although ultrasound is not always conclusive in diagnosing premature ovarian failure.

- **Genetic Testing**:
  In some cases, genetic testing may be recommended, especially if there is a family history of conditions like **Turner syndrome** or **fragile X syndrome**, which are associated with early ovarian failure.

Treatment Options and Fertility Preservation Strategies

While premature ovarian failure is often irreversible, there are treatment options and strategies that can help manage the symptoms and support fertility preservation. The approach to treatment depends on the individual's goals, whether that be managing symptoms of hormonal imbalance or seeking to preserve fertility.

1. **Hormone Replacement Therapy (HRT)**:

   One of the primary treatments for premature ovarian failure is **hormone replacement therapy** (HRT), which helps to restore estrogen and progesterone levels. HRT can relieve many of the symptoms associated with POF, such as hot flashes, night sweats, and mood swings. It also helps protect bone health and prevent osteoporosis. HRT is typically recommended until the woman reaches the typical age of menopause (around 50-51 years).

2. **Fertility Preservation**:

   For women with premature ovarian failure who wish to have children, fertility preservation techniques may be considered. The most effective method is **egg freezing (oocyte cryopreservation)**. If the ovaries are still producing some eggs, a woman can undergo hormonal stimulation to retrieve and freeze her eggs for future use. This process involves stimulating the ovaries with fertility drugs to produce multiple eggs, which are then harvested, frozen, and stored.

   - **Egg Donation**:

     For women with very little or no ovarian reserve, **egg donation** may be an option. This involves using eggs from a donor and fertilizing them with the partner's sperm. The resulting embryos can then be implanted into the woman's uterus.

3. **In Vitro Fertilization (IVF)**:

   In cases of premature ovarian failure, in vitro fertilization (IVF) using either the woman's own eggs (if available) or donor eggs is a viable fertility option. IVF involves fertilizing the eggs outside the body and then transferring the resulting embryos into the uterus.

4. **Alternative Therapies**:

   Some women may explore complementary therapies, such as acupuncture or herbal treatments, to support ovarian function or alleviate symptoms. While these therapies may provide symptomatic relief, they are generally not considered effective for reversing premature ovarian failure or restoring fertility.

5. **Psychological Support**:

   Experiencing premature ovarian failure can be emotionally challenging, especially for women who had hoped to conceive naturally. Psychological support through counseling or support groups can help women cope with the emotional toll of the condition. Fertility preservation options, though helpful, may not always guarantee success, and it is important to address the emotional aspects of living with POF.

Conclusion

Premature ovarian failure is a complex condition that can significantly affect a woman's fertility, hormonal health, and emotional well-being. While the exact cause of POF is often unknown, various factors, including genetic mutations, autoimmune disorders, and environmental exposures, can contribute to its development. Early diagnosis through blood tests and imaging can help women better understand their condition and plan for future fertility options.

While there is no cure for premature ovarian failure, treatment options, such as hormone replacement therapy, fertility preservation strategies, and IVF, can help women manage symptoms and increase their chances of having a biological child. For those who are not seeking to conceive, HRT can help maintain overall health and quality of life.

Premature ovarian failure is a journey that requires both medical intervention and emotional support. With the right care and resources, women can navigate this condition and achieve their reproductive and health goals.

Chapter 8

Female Infertility: Causes and Solutions

Introduction to Female Infertility

Infertility is a complex and often challenging condition that affects a significant number of couples globally. In approximately one-third of cases, infertility is due to female factors, one-third to male factors, and one-third to a combination of both or unexplained reasons. While infertility can be an emotionally difficult journey, it is important to remember that many women who struggle with infertility can successfully conceive with appropriate medical interventions, lifestyle adjustments, and emotional support.

Female infertility is typically defined as the inability to conceive after 12 months of regular, unprotected intercourse. However, for women over the age of 35, this time frame may be reduced to six months, as fertility tends to decline with age. The causes of female infertility are varied and can stem from issues with the ovaries, fallopian tubes, uterus, or hormonal regulation. Understanding the underlying causes and treatment options is crucial for women facing infertility, as it enables them to explore the right course of action for their reproductive health.

In this chapter, we will explore the common causes of female infertility, the diagnostic tests that can help identify these causes, and the available treatment options. Additionally, we will address the emotional impact of infertility and the support mechanisms that can assist women during this challenging experience.

Common Causes of Female Infertility

Female infertility can result from a variety of factors that disrupt the natural reproductive process. These factors may include problems with ovulation, blocked fallopian tubes, hormonal imbalances, or issues with the uterus. Let's take a closer look at the common causes of female infertility.

1. **Ovulatory Disorders**

The ovaries play a crucial role in fertility by producing and releasing eggs. Ovulatory disorders are one of the most common causes of female infertility. These disorders occur when a woman does not ovulate regularly or at all. Some of the most common ovulatory disorders include:

- **Polycystic Ovary Syndrome (PCOS)**: PCOS is one of the most prevalent causes of infertility in women. It is a hormonal disorder that leads to irregular periods, anovulation (lack of ovulation), and the development of multiple small cysts on the ovaries. Women with PCOS often have higher levels of androgens (male hormones), which can interfere with ovulation and lead to difficulty conceiving.

- **Hypothalamic Dysfunction**: The hypothalamus is a part of the brain that regulates the release of hormones necessary for ovulation. When the hypothalamus does not function properly, it can lead to irregular or absent ovulation. This condition can be caused by factors such as stress, excessive exercise, or eating disorders.

- **Premature Ovarian Insufficiency (POI)**: As discussed in the previous chapter, POI occurs when the ovaries stop functioning properly before the age of 40. Women with POI may experience a diminished ovarian reserve or no ovulation, making it difficult to conceive.

- **Luteal Phase Defect**: After ovulation, the body produces progesterone to support a potential pregnancy. A luteal phase defect occurs when the progesterone levels are insufficient to maintain the uterine lining for implantation, leading to early miscarriage or infertility.

2. **Blocked or Damaged Fallopian Tubes**

The fallopian tubes are essential for fertility as they provide the pathway for the egg to travel from the ovary to the uterus. If one or both fallopian tubes are blocked or damaged, it may prevent fertilization from occurring. The most common causes of fallopian tube damage or blockage include:

- **Pelvic Inflammatory Disease (PID)**: PID is a serious infection of the reproductive organs, often caused by sexually transmitted infections (STIs) such as chlamydia or gonorrhea. If left untreated, PID can lead to scarring and blockages in the fallopian tubes, making it difficult for the egg and sperm to meet.

- **Endometriosis**: Endometriosis is a condition in which tissue similar to the uterine lining grows outside the uterus, often affecting the ovaries and fallopian tubes. This tissue can cause scarring, adhesions, and blockages in the fallopian tubes, preventing egg fertilization.

- **Tubal Ligation**: Women who have undergone tubal ligation (a surgical procedure in which the fallopian tubes are cut or blocked) may experience infertility as a result of the blocked tubes. While tubal ligation is intended as a permanent form of birth control, some women may seek tubal reversal surgery to restore fertility.

3. **Hormonal Imbalances**

Hormonal imbalances can disrupt the normal reproductive process, leading to infertility. The hormones responsible for regulating the menstrual cycle, ovulation, and pregnancy include estrogen, progesterone, follicle-stimulating hormone (FSH), luteinizing hormone (LH), and prolactin. An imbalance in these hormones can affect ovulation, egg quality, and the ability to conceive.

- **Thyroid Disorders**: Both an overactive thyroid (hyperthyroidism) and an underactive thyroid (hypothyroidism) can disrupt the menstrual cycle and fertility. Thyroid hormones regulate many of the body's functions, including metabolism and reproductive health. Irregular thyroid levels can interfere with ovulation and the overall fertility process.
- **Hyperprolactinemia**: Prolactin is a hormone responsible for milk production after childbirth. However, excessive levels of prolactin (hyperprolactinemia) can disrupt normal menstrual cycles and prevent ovulation. This condition can be caused by various factors, including stress, medications, or pituitary gland abnormalities.

4. **Uterine and Cervical Issues**

The uterus is where the fertilized egg implants and grows during pregnancy. Conditions affecting the uterus can prevent pregnancy from occurring or cause complications after conception.

- **Uterine Fibroids**: Uterine fibroids are non-cancerous growths that develop in or around the uterus. Depending on their size and location, fibroids can block the fallopian tubes or interfere with implantation, leading to infertility or pregnancy loss.
- **Endometrial Polyps**: These are growths in the inner lining of the uterus (endometrium) that can interfere with embryo implantation. Endometrial polyps are often benign but can affect fertility.

- **Cervical Incompetence**: In some cases, a woman's cervix may not be able to support a pregnancy, leading to miscarriage or preterm birth. This condition may require treatment, such as a cervical cerclage (a stitch placed around the cervix), to prevent pregnancy loss.

5. **Age-Related Fertility Decline**

As women age, their fertility naturally declines due to a decrease in both the quantity and quality of eggs. A woman's peak reproductive years are typically in her late teens to late 20s, with fertility beginning to decline significantly after the age of 35. The decrease in egg quality, combined with a lower ovarian reserve, makes it more challenging to conceive as women get older. Additionally, older women are at a higher risk of miscarriage and chromosomal abnormalities, such as Down syndrome.

6. **Unexplained Infertility**

In some cases, no specific cause of infertility can be identified after a comprehensive evaluation. This is known as unexplained infertility, and it is relatively common, affecting about 20–30% of couples who have difficulty conceiving. While the cause remains elusive, treatment options such as in vitro fertilization (IVF) may still be successful in helping these couples achieve pregnancy.

Diagnostic Tests for Female Infertility

To determine the cause of infertility, healthcare providers typically begin with a thorough evaluation that includes a physical exam, medical history review, and a series of diagnostic tests. Common tests include:

1. **Blood Tests**:
   Blood tests can measure levels of reproductive hormones such as FSH, LH, estrogen, progesterone, and thyroid hormones. These tests help assess ovarian function, ovulation, and potential hormonal imbalances.

2. **Ultrasound**:
   A pelvic ultrasound can provide images of the ovaries, uterus, and fallopian tubes. This test can detect issues like ovarian cysts, uterine fibroids, or structural abnormalities in the reproductive organs.

3. **Hysterosalpingography (HSG)**:
   An HSG is an X-ray procedure that involves injecting dye into the uterus and fallopian tubes to check for blockages or abnormalities. It helps identify issues like blocked fallopian tubes or uterine abnormalities.

4. **Laparoscopy**:
   A laparoscopy is a minimally invasive surgical procedure used to examine the pelvic organs. It is often used to diagnose conditions such as endometriosis, fibroids, or pelvic adhesions that may be affecting fertility.

Treatment Options for Female Infertility

Depending on the cause of infertility, treatment options can range from lifestyle changes and medication to more advanced techniques like assisted reproductive technology (ART). Common treatments include:

1. **Lifestyle Modifications**:
   Lifestyle factors, such as maintaining a healthy weight, avoiding smoking and excessive alcohol, and reducing stress, can play a significant role in fertility. A well-balanced diet rich in nutrients, regular exercise, and

maintaining a healthy body mass index (BMI) can improve the chances of conception.

2. **Ovulation-Inducing Medications**:
   Medications like **clomiphene citrate** and **gonadotropins** are commonly prescribed to stimulate ovulation in women with ovulatory disorders like PCOS. These medications help encourage the release of eggs and can increase the chances of pregnancy, especially when combined with intrauterine insemination (IUI).

3. **In Vitro Fertilization (IVF)**:
   IVF is a highly effective treatment for infertility. In IVF, eggs are retrieved from the ovaries, fertilized in a laboratory, and then implanted into the uterus. IVF is often recommended for women with blocked fallopian tubes, severe male infertility, or unexplained infertility.

4. **Intrauterine Insemination (IUI)**:
   IUI involves placing sperm directly into the uterus around the time of ovulation. This treatment is often used in cases of mild male infertility or ovulatory disorders.

5. **Surgical Treatment**:
   In some cases, surgery may be necessary to correct anatomical issues such as blocked fallopian tubes, uterine fibroids, or endometriosis. Surgical procedures like laparoscopy can be used to remove fibroids, scar tissue, or adhesions to improve fertility.

6. **Egg or Embryo Donation**:
   For women with low ovarian reserve or premature ovarian failure, egg or

embryo donation may be an option. In this process, eggs from a donor are fertilized and implanted in the woman's uterus.

7. **Donor Sperm**:

   If male infertility is a factor, using donor sperm may be an option for women who are seeking pregnancy. Donor sperm is typically used in conjunction with IUI or IVF.

Emotional Impact and Support

Infertility is not only a physical challenge but also an emotional one. The journey of infertility can be emotionally draining, causing feelings of frustration, isolation, and sadness. Many women experience anxiety, depression, or a sense of loss as they navigate the uncertainty of whether or not they will ever have a biological child.

It is essential to address the emotional impact of infertility and seek support. Some strategies to help cope with the emotional challenges of infertility include:

- **Counseling and Therapy**: Professional counseling or therapy, either individually or with a partner, can provide emotional support and guidance. Cognitive-behavioral therapy (CBT) has been shown to help individuals cope with the stress and emotional strain of infertility.

- **Support Groups**: Joining a support group for women experiencing infertility can provide a sense of community and understanding. Connecting with others who are going through similar struggles can be reassuring and offer emotional validation.

- **Partner Support**: Infertility can place significant strain on relationships. Open communication, empathy, and shared decision-making are key to maintaining a strong partnership throughout the process. Couples may benefit from counseling to help strengthen their relationship during this challenging time.

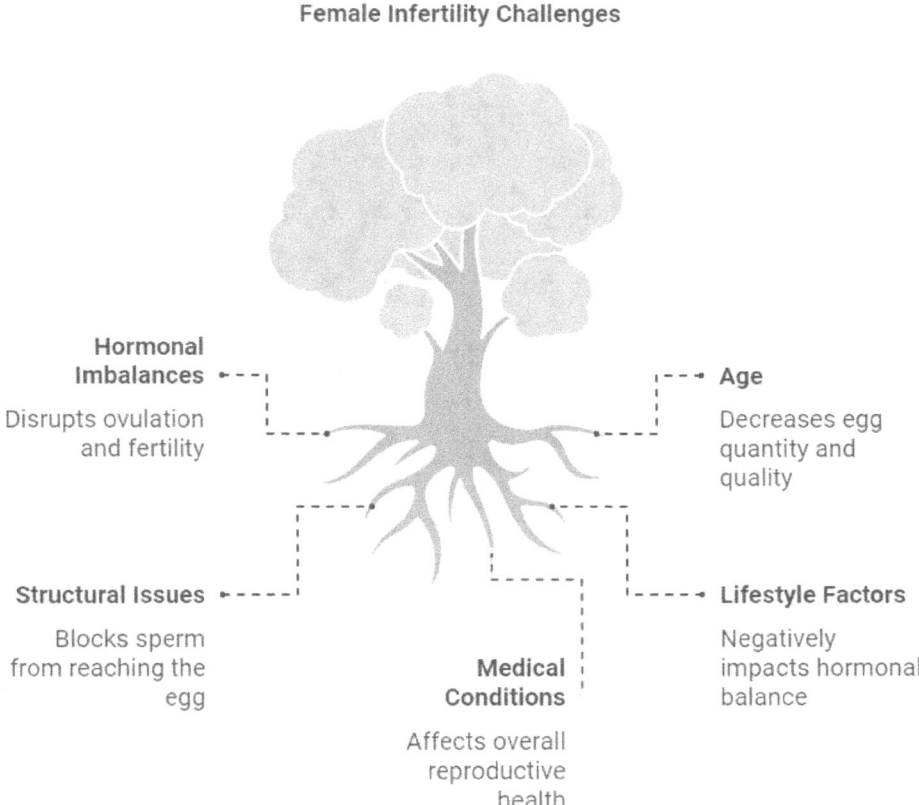

Conclusion

Female infertility is a multifaceted condition with a wide range of causes, from ovulatory disorders and blocked fallopian tubes to hormonal imbalances and age-related factors. Diagnostic tests are essential in identifying the underlying cause of infertility, and treatment options vary based on the specific diagnosis. These options may include lifestyle changes, medication, assisted reproductive technologies, and, in some cases, surgery.

While the path to conception can be difficult for many women, advances in fertility treatments have made it possible for many to achieve their dream of parenthood. The emotional impact of infertility should not be overlooked, and emotional support through counseling, support groups, and open communication with loved ones can help women cope with the challenges they face.

Infertility is a journey that requires both physical and emotional resilience. With the right support and medical care, many women can successfully overcome the challenges of infertility and build the families they have always envisioned.

Chapter 9

Introduction to Male Reproductive Health

The Male Reproductive System: Anatomy and Function

The male reproductive system is an intricate network of organs and glands that work together to produce, nourish, and deliver sperm. In addition to its primary role in reproduction, the male reproductive system also has critical functions in the production of male hormones, most notably testosterone. This chapter explores the anatomy of the male reproductive system and how its various components work together to facilitate reproduction.

The male reproductive system consists of both external and internal structures that play essential roles in the production and transport of sperm.

1. **External Organs**

- **Penis**: The penis is the external genital organ responsible for sexual intercourse and the expulsion of sperm. It has three primary components: the root (attached to the body), the shaft (the length of the penis), and the glans (the tip). The shaft contains erectile tissue, which fills with blood during sexual arousal, leading to an erection. The urethra, which runs through the center of the penis, allows for the passage of both urine and semen.

- **Scrotum**: The scrotum is a pouch of skin and muscle located beneath the penis that holds and protects the testicles. It is responsible for regulating the temperature of the testicles, as sperm production occurs most efficiently at a temperature slightly lower than body temperature. The scrotum can adjust its position to raise or lower the testicles, depending on the surrounding temperature, which helps to maintain optimal conditions for sperm production.

- **Testicles (Testes)**: The testicles are oval-shaped organs housed in the scrotum that are responsible for producing sperm and male hormones, including testosterone. Each testicle contains thousands of seminiferous tubules, where sperm production, or spermatogenesis, occurs. The testes also produce testosterone, the hormone responsible for the development of male characteristics such as facial hair, deep voice, and muscle mass.

2. **Internal Organs**

- **Epididymis**: Located behind each testicle, the epididymis is a long, coiled tube where sperm mature and are stored. Sperm undergo several stages of maturation in the epididymis before becoming capable of fertilizing an egg. This process takes about two to three weeks.

- **Vas Deferens**: The vas deferens is a muscular tube that transports mature sperm from the epididymis to the urethra in preparation for ejaculation. The vas deferens is a key component in the male reproductive system, as it ensures sperm travel efficiently from the site of production to the place where they are expelled from the body.

- **Seminal Vesicles**: These are small glands located behind the bladder that produce a significant portion of the semen. The seminal vesicles secrete a fluid rich in fructose and other substances that nourish and provide energy to sperm, facilitating their movement through the male reproductive tract and enhancing their chances of fertilizing an egg.

- **Prostate Gland**: The prostate is a walnut-sized gland located below the bladder. It produces a fluid that is essential for the semen's composition, helping to neutralize the acidic environment of the female reproductive tract, thus protecting sperm and enhancing their survival. The prostate also plays a role in the process of ejaculation.

- **Bulbourethral Glands (Cowper's Glands)**: These small glands, located near the base of the penis, secrete a clear, mucus-like fluid that helps lubricate the urethra during sexual activity and neutralizes any remaining acidity in the urethra, which could damage sperm.

- **Urethra**: The urethra is a tube that runs from the bladder to the penis and serves dual functions. It is responsible for the expulsion of both urine from the bladder and semen from the reproductive tract during ejaculation.

3. **Hormonal Regulation**

The production of sperm and male hormones is tightly regulated by hormones, primarily from the brain. The hypothalamus in the brain produces gonadotropin-releasing hormone (GnRH), which stimulates the pituitary gland to release two crucial hormones: follicle-stimulating hormone (FSH) and luteinizing hormone (LH).

- **FSH**: This hormone stimulates the testicles to produce sperm. It acts on the Sertoli cells within the seminiferous tubules, promoting sperm production (spermatogenesis).

- **LH**: LH stimulates the Leydig cells in the testicles to produce testosterone. This hormone is responsible for the development of male secondary sexual characteristics, including muscle mass, body hair, and deep voice. Testosterone also plays an essential role in the regulation of sperm production.

Testosterone, in turn, has numerous effects on the male body, from the development of reproductive tissues to maintaining bone density, red blood cell production, and mood regulation. The balance of these hormones ensures that the male reproductive system functions optimally.

Key Factors Affecting Male Reproductive Health

Male reproductive health is influenced by several factors that can affect the ability to produce healthy sperm and maintain sexual and hormonal balance. These factors include age, lifestyle choices, genetics, environmental influences, medical conditions, and psychological factors.

1. **Age and Fertility**

While fertility problems are often associated with women as they age, men's reproductive health also declines with age, albeit at a slower rate. Testosterone levels typically begin to decline around the age of 30, and sperm quality may decrease as men age, particularly after the age of 40. Older men may also experience a reduction in semen volume, sperm motility, and sperm concentration, all of which can contribute to difficulty in conception. Furthermore, advanced paternal age has been linked to an increased risk of certain genetic disorders in offspring, such as autism spectrum disorders and schizophrenia.

2. **Lifestyle Choices**

Certain lifestyle habits can significantly affect male reproductive health. These include:

- **Diet**: A poor diet high in processed foods, sugars, and unhealthy fats can negatively impact sperm quality. Conversely, a balanced diet rich in vitamins, antioxidants, and minerals, such as zinc, selenium, and folic acid, can enhance sperm count and motility.

- **Smoking**: Smoking has been shown to reduce sperm quality by decreasing sperm count, motility, and morphology (shape). It also increases the risk of erectile dysfunction and can have long-term effects on fertility.

- **Alcohol Consumption**: Excessive alcohol consumption can impair testosterone production and reduce sperm count and motility. It also increases the risk of erectile dysfunction and can contribute to other sexual health issues.

- **Substance Abuse**: The use of recreational drugs, such as marijuana, cocaine, and anabolic steroids, can have harmful effects on male fertility. These substances interfere with hormone production and sperm development, leading to low sperm counts and poor sperm quality.

- **Physical Activity**: Moderate physical activity is beneficial for overall health, including reproductive health. However, excessive exercise, especially in athletes or those who engage in high-intensity training, may reduce testosterone levels and negatively impact sperm production.

3. **Environmental Factors**

Environmental toxins and pollutants can also have a significant impact on male reproductive health. Exposure to certain chemicals, such as pesticides, heavy metals (e.g., lead and mercury), and endocrine-disrupting chemicals found in plastics and industrial products, can interfere with hormone production, sperm quality, and fertility. Additionally, exposure to high levels of heat, such as from hot tubs or frequent use of laptops on the lap, can raise the temperature of the testicles and negatively affect sperm production.

4. **Medical Conditions**

   Several medical conditions can affect male reproductive health, including:

   - **Varicocele**: A varicocele is an enlargement of the veins within the scrotum, which can lead to lower sperm quality by increasing the temperature in the testicles and reducing blood flow. It is one of the most common causes of male infertility and can often be corrected with surgery.

   - **Erectile Dysfunction (ED)**: Erectile dysfunction is a condition in which a man has difficulty achieving or maintaining an erection suitable for sexual intercourse. ED can result from physical causes, such as cardiovascular disease, diabetes, or nerve damage, or from psychological factors, including stress and anxiety. While ED is primarily a sexual health issue, it can also affect male fertility by preventing successful ejaculation and the delivery of sperm.

   - **Infections**: Infections of the reproductive system, such as sexually transmitted infections (STIs), can affect male fertility. Chlamydia, gonorrhea, and epididymitis can cause scarring or inflammation in the reproductive organs, which can reduce sperm quality or block sperm transport.

   - **Hormonal Imbalances**: Conditions like hypogonadism, where the body fails to produce enough testosterone, can lead to infertility by affecting sperm production and sexual function.

   - **Genetic Disorders**: Certain genetic disorders, such as Klinefelter syndrome (an extra X chromosome) or cystic fibrosis, can affect male fertility. These conditions can lead to low sperm count, infertility, or absent sperm.

5. **Psychological and Stress Factors**

Psychological factors, including stress, anxiety, and depression, can have a direct impact on male reproductive health. Chronic stress can interfere with hormone production, reduce sperm count, and impair sexual function. Furthermore, the emotional and mental toll of fertility challenges can exacerbate these issues, creating a cycle that may further complicate efforts to conceive.

6. **Medications and Treatments**

Certain medications and treatments can adversely affect male reproductive health. For example, chemotherapy, radiation therapy, and some medications used to treat conditions like high blood pressure, depression, and anxiety can have detrimental effects on sperm production. Men undergoing cancer treatment may experience temporary or permanent infertility, and in such cases, sperm banking for future use may be an option.

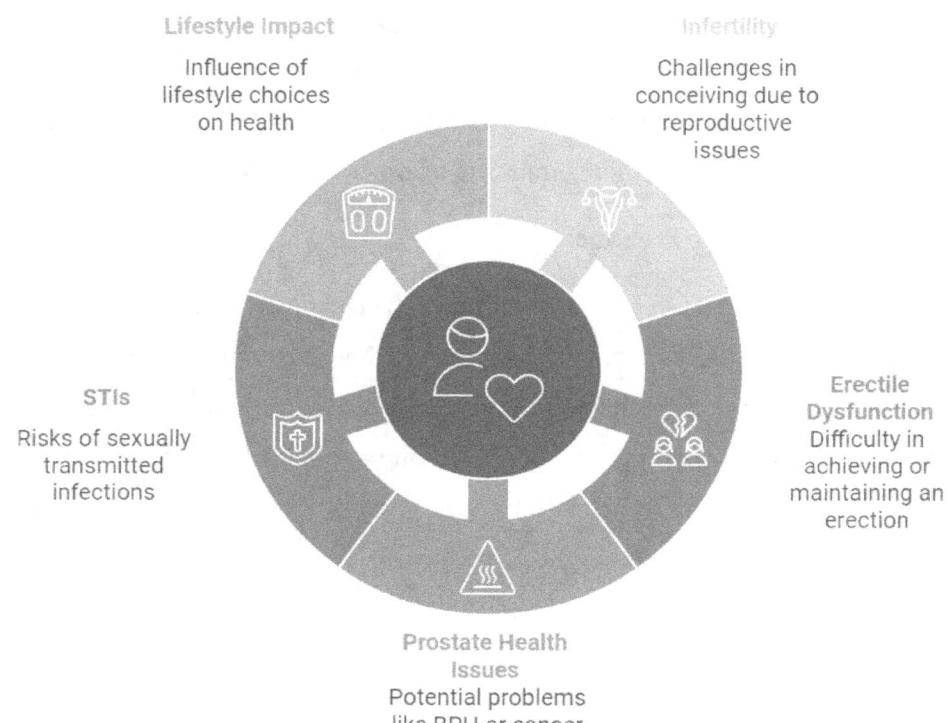

Conclusion

The male reproductive system is a complex and vital part of overall health and fertility. Understanding its anatomy and function, as well as the factors that affect male reproductive health, is crucial for addressing fertility issues and maintaining sexual well-being. Factors such as age, lifestyle choices, medical conditions, and environmental exposures can all play a significant role in male fertility. By recognizing and addressing these factors, men can take proactive steps to protect and enhance their reproductive health, leading to better fertility outcomes and overall health.

Chapter 10

Prostatitis: Understanding Symptoms and Treatment

What is Prostatitis and Its Causes?

Prostatitis is an inflammation of the prostate gland, a walnut-sized organ located below the bladder and in front of the rectum. The prostate's primary function is to produce a fluid that is a key component of semen, aiding in the nourishment and transport of sperm. Prostatitis can occur in men of all ages, but it is more common in men between the ages of 30 and 50.

The condition can range from mild to severe, and its causes can vary. Prostatitis may be due to bacterial infection, but it can also occur without any known infectious agent, which is referred to as nonbacterial prostatitis. The two main categories of prostatitis are acute prostatitis and chronic prostatitis, and each has distinct causes, symptoms, and treatment options.

Causes of Prostatitis

1. **Bacterial Infection**: One of the most common causes of prostatitis is a bacterial infection, often a result of bacteria entering the prostate through the urethra. The prostate gland may become infected by bacteria that originate from the bladder, urinary tract, or sexually transmitted infections (STIs) like gonorrhea or chlamydia. The infection can cause swelling, pain, and discomfort in the prostate, and in some cases, the infection may spread to other parts of the urinary tract, leading to more severe complications.

2. **Chronic Nonbacterial Prostatitis**: In some cases, prostatitis occurs without the presence of bacterial infection, and the cause remains unclear. This form of prostatitis is known as chronic nonbacterial prostatitis or chronic pelvic pain syndrome (CPPS). It is the most common form of prostatitis, and while

its exact cause is not fully understood, it is believed that factors such as stress, pelvic floor muscle tension, or nerve irritation may contribute to its development. Other possible factors include inflammation or autoimmune responses, which may result in the immune system attacking the prostate.

3. **Urinary Tract Infections (UTIs)**: UTIs, particularly when recurrent, can be a significant cause of bacterial prostatitis. The bacteria responsible for UTIs can migrate to the prostate, causing inflammation and infection.

4. **Prostate Stones**: In some men, small stones or calcifications can form in the prostate. These stones can irritate the prostate, potentially leading to an infection or contributing to chronic prostatitis.

5. **Sexually Transmitted Infections (STIs)**: Sexually transmitted infections such as gonorrhea and chlamydia are known to be potential causes of bacterial prostatitis. When left untreated, these infections can spread to the prostate and lead to significant inflammation.

6. **Trauma or Injury**: Any injury to the pelvic area or lower abdomen, such as from prolonged sitting, a sports injury, or a car accident, can cause trauma to the prostate and lead to prostatitis. In some cases, trauma to the perineum (the area between the genitals and anus) can also be a factor in the development of prostatitis.

7. **Immune System Dysfunction**: In rare cases, prostatitis can be linked to an abnormal immune system response, where the body's immune system mistakenly attacks the prostate tissue. This is typically associated with chronic prostatitis or chronic pelvic pain syndrome.

Symptoms of Prostatitis

The symptoms of prostatitis can vary greatly depending on the type of prostatitis and its underlying cause. Common symptoms include pain or discomfort in the pelvic region, urinary problems, and sexual dysfunction. While some men may experience only mild symptoms, others may have severe pain and discomfort that affects their quality of life.

1. **Painful Urination**: One of the hallmark symptoms of prostatitis is painful or burning urination. This discomfort occurs when the prostate becomes inflamed and presses on the urethra, making urination painful or difficult.

2. **Frequent Urination**: Men with prostatitis may experience the need to urinate frequently, especially during the night. This is often accompanied by an urgent need to urinate, even if the bladder is not full. This condition, known as nocturia, can interfere with sleep and cause significant discomfort.

3. **Pelvic or Lower Abdominal Pain**: Pain or discomfort in the pelvic region is common, particularly in the lower abdomen or groin area. Some men may also experience pain in the perineum (the area between the genitals and anus), lower back, or genital region. The pain may be sharp or aching and can vary in intensity.

4. **Painful Ejaculation**: Men with prostatitis often report pain or discomfort during or after ejaculation. This is a particularly distressing symptom for many men, as it can affect their sexual health and relationships.

5. **Pain in the Lower Back or Groin**: Chronic prostatitis may cause persistent or intermittent pain in the lower back, groin, or perineum. This pain is usually dull and achy, but it can become sharper during sexual activity or when sitting for extended periods.

6. **Flu-like Symptoms**: Acute bacterial prostatitis can lead to systemic symptoms such as fever, chills, nausea, and malaise (general feeling of discomfort or illness). These symptoms indicate the presence of an infection and may require immediate medical attention.

7. **Sexual Dysfunction**: Prostatitis can contribute to erectile dysfunction (ED), which is difficulty achieving or maintaining an erection. The pain associated with prostatitis can also affect libido and sexual desire, further complicating sexual health.

8. **Blood in Urine or Semen**: In more severe cases of prostatitis, blood may appear in the urine or semen. This is typically a sign of inflammation or infection and should be evaluated by a healthcare professional.

Types of Prostatitis

1. **Acute Bacterial Prostatitis**: This is a severe, sudden-onset infection of the prostate gland caused by bacteria. It is considered a medical emergency and requires immediate treatment. Symptoms include high fever, chills, painful urination, pelvic pain, and general body discomfort. If left untreated, acute bacterial prostatitis can lead to complications such as abscess formation, septicemia (infection in the bloodstream), or kidney damage.

2. **Chronic Bacterial Prostatitis**: This type of prostatitis is a less common, persistent infection that lasts for at least three months. It is usually caused by the same bacteria responsible for acute bacterial prostatitis, but the infection may be less severe and more difficult to treat. Symptoms of chronic bacterial prostatitis include frequent urination, pelvic pain, and painful ejaculation. Chronic bacterial prostatitis can be challenging to treat, as bacteria often

hide within prostate tissue, making it hard for antibiotics to completely eradicate the infection.

3. **Chronic Nonbacterial Prostatitis (Chronic Pelvic Pain Syndrome)**: This is the most common type of prostatitis and is not caused by bacterial infection. Men with chronic nonbacterial prostatitis often experience chronic pelvic pain, painful urination, and sexual dysfunction. The cause of this condition is not fully understood, and it is thought to result from factors such as pelvic floor muscle dysfunction, nerve sensitivity, or psychological stress. Although bacterial infections are ruled out, inflammation remains present in the prostate.

4. **Asymptomatic Inflammatory Prostatitis**: This form of prostatitis does not cause noticeable symptoms, and many men are unaware they have it. Asymptomatic inflammatory prostatitis is often discovered incidentally during routine medical exams or tests for other conditions. While it may not require immediate treatment, it can sometimes be linked to fertility problems.

Treatment Options for Prostatitis

Treatment for prostatitis depends on the type of prostatitis, the underlying cause, and the severity of symptoms. A healthcare provider will conduct a thorough evaluation to determine the most appropriate treatment plan.

1. **Antibiotics**: For bacterial prostatitis, antibiotics are the primary treatment. In cases of acute bacterial prostatitis, intravenous (IV) antibiotics may be necessary to quickly reduce the infection. For chronic bacterial prostatitis, a longer course of oral antibiotics may be required, sometimes for several weeks or even months. It is essential to complete the entire course of

antibiotics, even if symptoms improve, to ensure the infection is fully eradicated.

2. **Pain Management**: Pain relief is a crucial part of prostatitis treatment, especially for those experiencing significant discomfort. Over-the-counter (OTC) pain relievers such as ibuprofen, acetaminophen, or aspirin may help reduce inflammation and relieve pain. For more severe pain, a healthcare provider may prescribe stronger medications, including prescription painkillers or muscle relaxants, to ease pelvic floor tension and reduce spasms.

3. **Alpha-Blockers**: Alpha-blockers are medications that help relax the muscles around the prostate and bladder neck, making it easier to urinate. These medications can be particularly helpful for men experiencing urinary symptoms such as painful urination or frequent urination.

4. **Lifestyle Modifications**: Certain lifestyle changes can help reduce the symptoms of prostatitis and prevent flare-ups. Recommendations include:
   - **Dietary Adjustments**: Avoiding spicy foods, caffeine, and alcohol, which can irritate the bladder and prostate.
   - **Hydration**: Drinking plenty of water can help flush out bacteria and toxins from the urinary tract.
   - **Regular Exercise**: Engaging in regular physical activity, particularly pelvic floor exercises, can help relieve pelvic pain and improve overall prostate health.

    - **Stress Management**: Reducing stress through relaxation techniques, such as deep breathing, meditation, or yoga, can alleviate the symptoms of chronic prostatitis.
5. **Surgical Interventions**: In rare cases, surgical treatment may be necessary, especially if an abscess (a collection of pus) forms in the prostate or if there are complications such as prostate stones. Surgical procedures can also help if prostatitis is causing significant blockages in the urinary tract.
6. **Psychological Therapy**: For chronic nonbacterial prostatitis, managing psychological factors such as stress, anxiety, or depression can be crucial. Cognitive behavioral therapy (CBT) and other forms of psychotherapy may help men cope with the chronic pain and emotional distress associated with the condition.

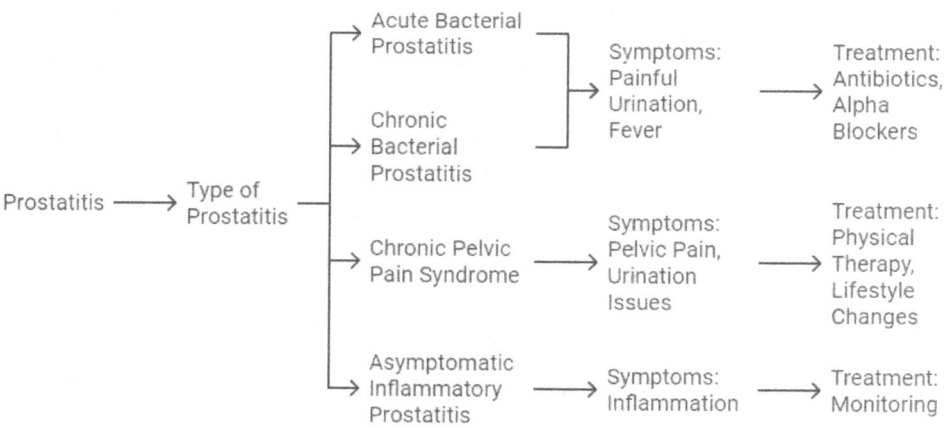

Conclusion

Prostatitis is a condition that can have a significant impact on a man's health and well-being. Understanding the different types of prostatitis, their causes, and the available treatment options is key to managing the symptoms and improving quality of life. While bacterial prostatitis is typically treated with antibiotics, other forms of prostatitis, such as chronic nonbacterial prostatitis, require a more comprehensive approach that includes pain management, lifestyle changes, and sometimes psychological support. With appropriate care and treatment, men with prostatitis can manage their symptoms and return to normal, active lives.

Chapter 11

Male Infertility: Identifying and Overcoming Challenges

Introduction to Male Infertility

Male infertility refers to the inability of a man to contribute to conception, despite having regular unprotected sexual intercourse. This condition is a complex issue, involving various biological, environmental, and lifestyle factors that can hinder the production of healthy sperm or impair their ability to reach and fertilize an egg. Infertility in men is more common than many realize, affecting about 1 in 10 men globally. However, male infertility is often underreported and underdiscussed, partially due to societal stigmas and a lack of awareness.

Infertility affects not only the individual's physical health but also their emotional and psychological well-being. Understanding the causes, diagnostic tests, and available treatments for male infertility can help men navigate this challenging journey. In this chapter, we will delve into the common causes of male infertility, diagnostic tests used to assess fertility, treatment options available, and the emotional impact that infertility can have on men.

Common Causes of Male Infertility

Several factors contribute to male infertility, ranging from issues with sperm production to problems with sperm function or delivery. Male infertility can be categorized into several broad groups based on the underlying cause: problems with sperm production, sperm transport, and the surrounding environment.

1. **Sperm Production Issues (Low Sperm Count or Poor Sperm Quality)**

One of the most common causes of male infertility is a low sperm count (oligospermia), where the number of sperm in the semen is insufficient for conception. Additionally, poor sperm quality (e.g., poor motility or morphology) can further hinder the ability of sperm to fertilize an egg.

Azoospermia refers to the complete absence of sperm in the semen, which may be caused by a variety of factors, including genetic disorders, obstructions in the reproductive system, or issues with sperm production in the testes.

The following conditions can lead to sperm production issues:

- **Varicocele**: This condition, characterized by swollen veins in the scrotum, can interfere with sperm production by increasing the temperature around the testes.
- **Hormonal Imbalances**: Hormones regulate sperm production. Disorders involving the hypothalamus, pituitary gland, or testes can result in a lower sperm count or poor sperm quality.
- **Genetic Disorders**: Chromosomal abnormalities such as Klinefelter syndrome (where a male has an extra X chromosome) can result in impaired sperm production or even azoospermia.
- **Infections**: Some infections, such as mumps, sexually transmitted infections (STIs), or inflammation of the prostate, can affect sperm production.

2. **Sperm Transport Issues (Blockages or Structural Abnormalities)**

Male infertility can also arise from structural issues that block or impede the movement of sperm. A blockage or obstruction in the male reproductive tract prevents sperm from reaching the semen during ejaculation, thus hindering the fertilization process.

Possible causes include:

- **Vasectomy**: A vasectomy is a common surgical procedure in which the vas deferens (the tubes that carry sperm from the testes to the urethra) are cut or sealed. Though it is a highly effective form of contraception, it can cause permanent infertility unless reversed.

- **Congenital Abnormalities**: Some men are born with congenital abnormalities that affect the reproductive system, such as a missing or malformed vas deferens. Cystic fibrosis, a genetic disorder, is one example of a condition that can cause such abnormalities.

- **Infections or Inflammation**: Infections such as epididymitis or prostatitis can lead to scarring and blockage of the tubes that carry sperm, obstructing sperm transport.

3. **Ejaculation Disorders**

Even when sperm is produced in adequate quantities and is healthy, issues related to ejaculation can still result in infertility. In cases of **retrograde ejaculation**, sperm enters the bladder instead of being expelled through the urethra, which significantly reduces the chances of conception. This can occur as a result of nerve damage, diabetes, or surgery.

4. **Environmental and Lifestyle Factors**

Environmental and lifestyle factors play a significant role in male fertility. Modern-day environmental pollutants, chemical exposures, and unhealthy lifestyle habits can negatively affect sperm production and quality. These factors include:

- **Exposure to Toxins and Chemicals**: Long-term exposure to pesticides, heavy metals, and industrial chemicals has been linked to a decrease in sperm count and quality.

- **Heat Exposure**: Prolonged exposure to high temperatures (such as using hot tubs, saunas, or wearing tight-fitting clothing) can affect sperm production. The testes are located outside the body to keep the sperm cooler than the body's core temperature, and excessive heat can impair sperm production.
- **Smoking**: Cigarette smoking is associated with lower sperm count, reduced sperm motility, and changes in sperm morphology.
- **Alcohol and Drug Use**: Excessive alcohol consumption and illicit drug use (such as marijuana or anabolic steroids) can significantly reduce sperm production and quality.
- **Obesity**: Excess body weight can lead to hormonal imbalances and decreased sperm quality, as well as impair overall fertility.
- **Stress**: Chronic stress can negatively impact fertility by affecting hormone production, reducing libido, and leading to other health problems that hinder sperm production.

5. **Age-Related Decline in Fertility**

While male fertility does not experience the same sharp decline as female fertility with age, it does decrease gradually. As men age, sperm motility, morphology, and overall sperm quality may deteriorate, making it more difficult to conceive. Men over the age of 40 may also experience a decline in testosterone levels, which can further impair fertility.

Diagnostic Tests for Male Infertility

To diagnose male infertility, doctors typically begin with a detailed medical history, physical examination, and semen analysis. Several diagnostic tests can help identify the underlying cause of infertility:

1. **Semen Analysis**: The primary diagnostic test for male infertility is semen analysis, which assesses sperm count, motility (movement), morphology (shape), and overall semen volume. This test helps determine whether sperm production or quality is the issue.

2. **Blood Tests**: Blood tests can measure hormone levels, including testosterone, follicle-stimulating hormone (FSH), luteinizing hormone (LH), and prolactin. These tests help identify hormonal imbalances that may affect sperm production.

3. **Ultrasound**: A scrotal ultrasound may be used to detect any abnormalities in the testes or vas deferens, such as varicoceles, cysts, or blockages that could affect sperm production or transport.

4. **Genetic Testing**: Genetic tests can identify chromosomal abnormalities, such as Klinefelter syndrome or Y chromosome microdeletions, that may be contributing to male infertility.

5. **Post-Ejaculation Urine Analysis**: For men who may have retrograde ejaculation, a urine analysis after ejaculation can check for sperm in the urine. This helps diagnose the condition and identify potential treatment options.

6. **Testicular Biopsy**: In cases of azoospermia (no sperm in the semen), a testicular biopsy can determine whether sperm production is occurring in the testes. This test can also help doctors determine whether sperm retrieval is possible for assisted reproductive techniques like in vitro fertilization (IVF).

Treatment Options for Male Infertility

Once the cause of infertility is identified, several treatment options are available to address the condition and improve the chances of conception.

1. **Medications**:
   - **Hormonal Treatments**: If hormonal imbalances are identified as the cause of infertility, medications like gonadotropins or clomiphene citrate can stimulate sperm production. In cases of low testosterone, testosterone replacement therapy may be recommended.
   - **Antibiotics**: If an infection is found to be affecting sperm quality or production, antibiotics may be prescribed to treat the underlying infection.

2. **Surgical Treatments**:
   - **Varicocele Repair**: If varicoceles (swollen veins) are causing reduced sperm count, surgery can repair the veins and restore normal sperm production.
   - **Vasectomy Reversal**: In cases where a vasectomy has been performed and a man wishes to reverse the procedure, surgery can reconnect the vas deferens to restore sperm transport.

3. **Assisted Reproductive Technologies (ART)**: If sperm production is not sufficient, ART procedures such as intrauterine insemination (IUI) or in vitro fertilization (IVF) can be used. In these treatments, sperm is collected, concentrated, and then placed directly into the woman's reproductive system, or fertilization occurs outside the body, with the fertilized embryo being implanted into the uterus.

4. **Sperm Retrieval**: For men with azoospermia, sperm can sometimes be directly extracted from the testes using methods such as testicular sperm extraction (TESE). The retrieved sperm can then be used for IVF or ICSI (intracytoplasmic sperm injection), a procedure where a single sperm is injected into an egg.

5. **Lifestyle Changes**: Men experiencing infertility are often encouraged to adopt healthier lifestyle habits, such as:
    - Quitting smoking.
    - Limiting alcohol consumption.
    - Maintaining a healthy weight.
    - Managing stress.
    - Avoiding heat exposure to the testes.

Emotional and Psychological Impact of Male Infertility

The emotional toll of male infertility can be significant, often leading to feelings of inadequacy, frustration, guilt, and anxiety. Unlike female infertility, which is often more visible and openly discussed, male infertility is often shrouded in silence, contributing to emotional isolation. Many men may feel embarrassed or reluctant to seek help, which can lead to relationship strain, mental health issues, and a diminished sense of self-worth.

Infertility treatment can also be emotionally taxing, with the pressure of medical procedures, the uncertainty of success, and the possibility of failure. Men may experience stress, depression, or even resentment towards their partners or themselves as they navigate these challenges.

Psychological counseling, couples therapy, and support groups for men dealing with infertility can provide essential support and coping strategies. Open communication between partners is crucial for managing the emotional aspects of infertility, helping both individuals support each other and share their concerns.

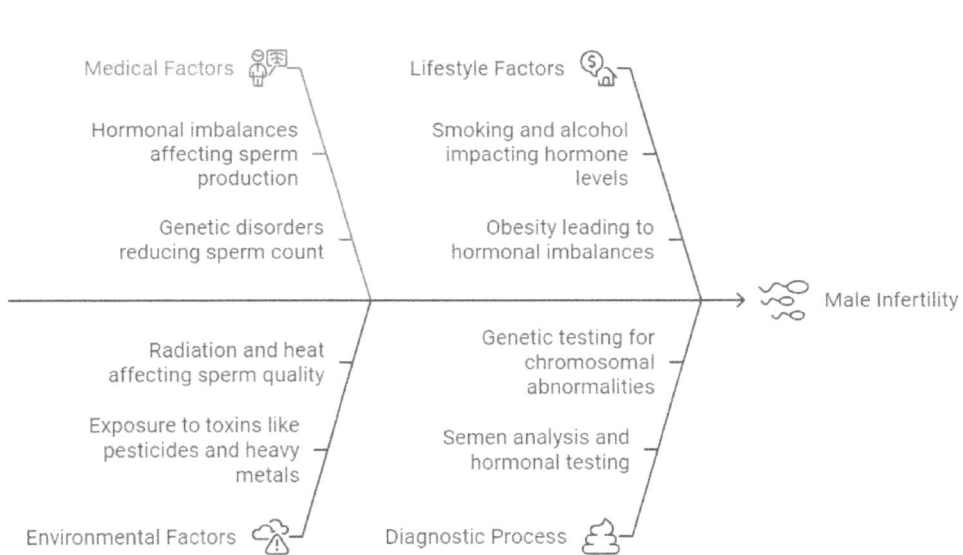

Conclusion

Male infertility is a multifaceted condition with various causes, from low sperm count to hormonal imbalances and structural issues in the reproductive system. With advancements in diagnostic techniques and treatment options, many men are able to overcome these challenges and become fathers. Understanding the causes, treatments, and emotional impact of male infertility is essential for men who are facing this issue. By seeking proper medical care, making lifestyle changes, and addressing the psychological aspects of infertility, men can navigate this journey with hope and confidence.

Chapter 12

Introduction to STIs: Prevention and Awareness

Understanding Sexually Transmitted Infections (STIs)

Sexually transmitted infections (STIs) are infections that are passed from one person to another through sexual contact. These infections can affect various parts of the body, but are most commonly associated with the genital area, mouth, and throat. STIs are a significant public health concern worldwide, as they can lead to serious reproductive health issues, increased risk of acquiring other infections, and in some cases, long-term health complications if left untreated.

The World Health Organization (WHO) estimates that more than 1 million STIs are acquired every day worldwide. Despite the alarming prevalence of these infections, many individuals are unaware of their risk factors, symptoms, or the potential long-term consequences of untreated STIs. A key challenge in the fight against STIs is the stigma surrounding them, which can prevent individuals from seeking testing, treatment, and discussing their sexual health openly with healthcare providers or partners.

This chapter provides an overview of the most common STIs, their impact on reproductive health, as well as practical guidance on prevention, testing, and the importance of communication between partners. Knowledge and awareness are vital tools in reducing the spread of STIs, improving sexual health, and protecting reproductive function.

Common STIs and Their Impact on Reproductive Health

Several types of STIs are prevalent across the globe, each with different modes of transmission, symptoms, and potential long-term consequences. While many STIs are treatable with antibiotics or antiviral medications, others can lead to chronic health issues if left untreated. Below are some of the most common STIs and their potential impact on reproductive health.

1. **Chlamydia**

    Cause: Chlamydia is a bacterial infection caused by *Chlamydia trachomatis*.

    Transmission: This infection is primarily transmitted through vaginal, anal, or oral sex. It can also be passed from mother to baby during childbirth.

    Symptoms: Chlamydia is often asymptomatic, meaning that many individuals may not experience any noticeable symptoms. When symptoms do occur, they may include abnormal discharge, pain during urination, and pelvic pain in women, and testicular pain or swelling in men.

    Reproductive Health Impact: Untreated chlamydia can lead to pelvic inflammatory disease (PID) in women, which can cause chronic pain, scarring, and infertility. In men, it can lead to epididymitis, an inflammation of the tubes that carry sperm, which can affect fertility.

2. **Gonorrhea**

    Cause: Gonorrhea is a bacterial infection caused by *Neisseria gonorrhoeae*.

    Transmission: Gonorrhea is transmitted through sexual contact with an infected person. It can also be passed from mother to baby during childbirth.

    Symptoms: Like chlamydia, gonorrhea may not cause symptoms in many people. When symptoms do occur, they can include painful urination, abnormal discharge, and pelvic pain. Men may experience pain or swelling in the testicles.

    Reproductive Health Impact: If left untreated, gonorrhea can also lead to PID in women, increasing the risk of infertility. In men, untreated gonorrhea can lead to complications such as prostatitis or infertility. Gonorrhea infections can also make individuals more susceptible to HIV.

3. **Human Immunodeficiency Virus (HIV)**

Cause: HIV is a virus that attacks the immune system, specifically targeting CD4 cells (T cells), which are essential for immune function.

Transmission: HIV is primarily transmitted through blood, semen, vaginal fluids, and breast milk. It is most commonly spread through unprotected sexual intercourse and sharing needles.

Symptoms: Early symptoms of HIV may resemble the flu or cold, including fever, sore throat, and swollen lymph nodes. As the infection progresses, individuals may develop AIDS (Acquired Immunodeficiency Syndrome), a severe weakening of the immune system.

Reproductive Health Impact: HIV does not directly affect reproductive organs but can lead to complications in pregnancy and childbirth. Pregnant women with untreated HIV can transmit the virus to their child, either during pregnancy, delivery, or breastfeeding. HIV also increases the risk of contracting other STIs, which can, in turn, affect fertility and reproductive health.

4. **Herpes Simplex Virus (HSV)**

Cause: Herpes is caused by the herpes simplex virus, with two types: HSV-1 (commonly causes oral herpes) and HSV-2 (commonly causes genital herpes).

Transmission: Herpes is spread through direct contact with infected skin, mucous membranes, or bodily fluids. This can occur through vaginal, anal, or oral sex, or even through casual skin-to-skin contact.

Symptoms: Herpes causes painful blisters or sores on the genital, anal, or oral areas. However, many people with herpes may not experience symptoms or may have only mild ones. The virus remains in the body, lying dormant in nerve cells, and can reactivate at any time.

Reproductive Health Impact: Genital herpes can cause painful outbreaks and complications during pregnancy. If a woman has an active outbreak during delivery, there is a risk of passing the virus to the newborn, which can cause severe health issues. In rare cases, repeated outbreaks can affect fertility.

5. **Human Papillomavirus (HPV)**

Cause: HPV is a group of more than 200 related viruses, some of which can cause genital warts and are associated with several cancers, including cervical, anal, and throat cancer.

Transmission: HPV is primarily transmitted through sexual contact, including vaginal, anal, and oral sex.

Symptoms: Many types of HPV cause no symptoms and resolve on their own. However, some strains lead to genital warts, while others may cause abnormal changes to cervical cells that can lead to cervical cancer.

Reproductive Health Impact: High-risk strains of HPV can cause cervical dysplasia (precancerous changes in cervical cells), which may eventually develop into cervical cancer if not treated. Regular screening with Pap smears and HPV tests are essential for early detection and prevention of cervical cancer.

6. **Syphilis**

Cause: Syphilis is a bacterial infection caused by *Treponema pallidum.*

Transmission: It is transmitted through direct contact with syphilitic sores during vaginal, anal, or oral sex. It can also be passed from mother to baby during pregnancy (congenital syphilis).

Symptoms: Syphilis typically progresses in four stages: primary, secondary, latent, and tertiary. The primary stage presents as a painless sore or ulcer, usually on the genitals, anus, or mouth. In the secondary stage, individuals may experience a rash, swollen lymph nodes, and flu-like symptoms. If left untreated, syphilis can progress to more severe stages, leading to organ damage and even death.

Reproductive Health Impact: Untreated syphilis can cause infertility, particularly if the infection reaches the tertiary stage, where it can damage vital organs. Syphilis can also increase the risk of HIV transmission. Congenital syphilis can lead to miscarriage, stillbirth, or severe birth defects.

Prevention of STIs

The best way to protect oneself and one's partner from STIs is through prevention. Several strategies can reduce the risk of acquiring or transmitting STIs:

1. **Condom Use**: The consistent and correct use of condoms (male or female) during all forms of sexual activity is one of the most effective ways to reduce the risk of STIs. Condoms act as a barrier to prevent direct contact with bodily fluids and infected areas of the body.

2. **Vaccination**: Vaccines are available for certain STIs, such as the HPV vaccine and the hepatitis B vaccine. Vaccination can significantly reduce the risk of infection and its associated health complications, including cancer.

3. **Regular Testing**: Regular STI screenings are essential for sexually active individuals, especially for those with multiple partners or unprotected sex.

Early detection allows for prompt treatment and reduces the risk of complications.

4. **Mutual Monogamy**: Being in a mutually monogamous relationship, where both partners are uninfected and have no other sexual partners, reduces the risk of STIs. It is crucial for both partners to communicate openly about their sexual health and undergo regular screenings.

5. **Avoiding Risky Behaviors**: Limiting the number of sexual partners and avoiding risky behaviors, such as sharing needles or having unprotected sex with high-risk individuals, can reduce exposure to STIs.

6. **Partner Communication**: Open, honest communication with sexual partners about sexual history, STI testing, and condom use is key to preventing the spread of infections. It is important to discuss any potential risks and mutual health concerns before engaging in sexual activity.

Comprehensive STI Awareness and Prevention

Importance of Awareness
Role of education and awareness in STI prevention

Definition of STIs
Understanding what STIs are and their causes

Prevention Strategies
Methods to prevent the spread of STIs

Symptoms
Common signs and symptoms of STIs

Conclusion

STIs are a widespread health concern with the potential to significantly impact reproductive health and overall well-being. Many STIs are treatable, and with proper prevention measures, the risks of transmission can be significantly reduced. Awareness, regular testing, communication with sexual partners, and practicing safe sex are essential steps in minimizing the impact of STIs on sexual and reproductive health. By taking proactive measures, individuals can maintain their health, prevent the spread of infections, and ensure a safer sexual experience for themselves and their partners.

Chapter 13

Genital Herpes: Myths, Facts, and Management

Understanding Herpes Simplex Virus (HSV)

Genital herpes is a common sexually transmitted infection (STI) caused by the herpes simplex virus (HSV). HSV comes in two forms: HSV-1 and HSV-2. While both types can cause genital herpes, HSV-2 is typically responsible for most genital infections, whereas HSV-1 is most commonly associated with oral herpes, which causes cold sores. However, HSV-1 can also cause genital herpes through oral-genital contact, making it important to understand the distinction between the two and their potential impact on sexual health.

Herpes simplex viruses are highly contagious and can remain dormant in the body for long periods, occasionally reactivating to cause outbreaks. The virus primarily affects the skin and mucous membranes, particularly in the genital and anal regions. It is crucial to understand how HSV spreads, its symptoms, and the available treatments to manage outbreaks effectively.

Despite its prevalence, there are many misconceptions surrounding genital herpes. In this chapter, we will break down common myths, present facts, and explore the options available for managing and living with the condition.

Symptoms, Transmission, and Risk Factors

1. **Symptoms of Genital Herpes**

The symptoms of genital herpes can vary greatly from person to person. Many individuals infected with HSV may not experience any symptoms or may have very mild symptoms that are easily overlooked. However, for those who do experience symptoms, they can include:

- **Painful Sores**: The most common symptom of genital herpes is the appearance of painful blisters or sores in the genital, anal, or surrounding areas. These blisters may rupture, leaving open ulcers that can be painful, especially during urination.

- **Itching or Tingling Sensations**: Many people report itching, tingling, or a burning sensation in the affected area, even before visible sores appear. These sensations are often referred to as "prodromal symptoms" and can serve as an early warning of an impending outbreak.

- **Flu-like Symptoms**: In some cases, especially during the first outbreak, individuals may experience fever, body aches, swollen lymph nodes, and a headache, similar to flu symptoms.

- **Painful Urination**: When sores are present near the genital or anal areas, urination can be painful due to the irritation caused by the sores.

The first outbreak of genital herpes is often the most severe, and subsequent outbreaks are typically less intense. However, the virus can remain dormant in the body and reactivate later, particularly during times of stress, illness, or a weakened immune system.

2. **Transmission of Genital Herpes**

HSV is primarily transmitted through direct skin-to-skin contact, most commonly during vaginal, anal, or oral sex. It can also be transmitted when there are no visible symptoms, which makes the virus difficult to detect and prevent. Here are the key modes of transmission:

- **Sexual Contact**: Genital herpes can be transmitted through vaginal, anal, or oral sex with an infected partner, even if the infected person is not showing symptoms. The virus is present in the fluid of the blisters, as well as in saliva and genital secretions.
- **Skin-to-Skin Contact**: Herpes can also spread through close contact with infected skin, even if there are no visible sores present. This means it is possible to contract the virus through genital contact, even if no symptoms are apparent at the time.
- **Mother to Child**: Pregnant women with active genital herpes are at risk of transmitting the virus to their baby during delivery. This is known as neonatal herpes and can lead to severe complications for the newborn. It is crucial for pregnant women to discuss their herpes status with their healthcare provider to determine the best approach during delivery.

Risk Factors for Genital Herpes:

- **Unprotected Sexual Activity**: The risk of contracting HSV is higher when engaging in unprotected sexual activity, especially with multiple sexual partners or if a partner has an active outbreak.
- **Weakened Immune System**: People with weakened immune systems, such as those with HIV/AIDS, may be more susceptible to contracting and experiencing more frequent outbreaks of genital herpes.
- **Previous STIs**: Those who have had other sexually transmitted infections (STIs), such as chlamydia or gonorrhea, are at increased

risk of contracting genital herpes because the presence of another infection can make the skin more vulnerable to viral entry.

- **Early Sexual Activity**: Individuals who begin sexual activity at an early age are at a higher risk of contracting genital herpes, as they may have had greater exposure to unprotected sex.

Myths and Facts About Genital Herpes

There are many myths about genital herpes that can cause unnecessary fear and misinformation. It is important to separate fact from fiction to better understand the infection and reduce the stigma associated with it.

1. **Myth**: Genital herpes is rare.
    - **Fact**: Genital herpes is extremely common. It is estimated that nearly 1 in 6 people in the United States between the ages of 14 and 49 have genital herpes, and the prevalence is similar worldwide. Many people who are infected do not show symptoms, contributing to the spread of the virus.

2. **Myth**: You can only get herpes if you have visible sores.
    - **Fact**: It is possible to contract genital herpes even if the infected person does not have visible sores or any symptoms. This is known as "asymptomatic shedding," where the virus is present in the skin and genital fluids but does not produce noticeable symptoms.

3. **Myth**: Genital herpes is a lifelong sentence of constant outbreaks.
    - **Fact**: While there is currently no cure for herpes, most people experience only occasional outbreaks, and the frequency of outbreaks tends to decrease over time. With proper management, many

individuals with genital herpes can live symptom-free and lead normal, healthy lives.

4. **Myth**: People with herpes can't have normal relationships.
   - **Fact**: People with genital herpes can have healthy, fulfilling relationships. With open communication, appropriate precautions, and treatment, individuals with herpes can have satisfying sexual relationships and reduce the risk of transmission.

Treatment and Strategies for Managing Outbreaks

While there is no cure for genital herpes, there are several ways to manage the infection and reduce the frequency and severity of outbreaks. The goal of treatment is to minimize symptoms, prevent the spread of the virus, and improve the quality of life for individuals living with the infection.

1. **Antiviral Medications**: The primary treatment for genital herpes is antiviral medication. These medications help to control the virus, shorten the duration of outbreaks, and reduce the likelihood of transmission to others. Some commonly prescribed antiviral medications for herpes include:
   - **Acyclovir** (Zovirax)
   - **Valacyclovir** (Valtrex)
   - **Famciclovir** (Famvir)

These medications can be taken during an outbreak (episodic treatment) or daily as suppressive therapy to prevent outbreaks from occurring (suppressive treatment). Daily antiviral treatment has been shown to significantly reduce the frequency of outbreaks and lower the risk of transmitting the virus to others.

2. **Pain Relief**: Pain management is an important part of treating genital herpes, especially during an outbreak. Over-the-counter pain relievers, such as ibuprofen or acetaminophen, can help reduce pain and inflammation. Additionally, applying cool compresses to the affected area or using numbing creams may provide some relief from discomfort.

3. **Lifestyle Adjustments**: Certain lifestyle changes can help reduce the frequency of outbreaks and support overall health. These include:

    - **Reducing Stress**: Stress is a known trigger for herpes outbreaks. Practicing relaxation techniques, such as meditation, yoga, or deep breathing exercises, can help manage stress and reduce the likelihood of outbreaks.

    - **Maintaining a Healthy Immune System**: A strong immune system can help the body suppress the virus. Eating a balanced diet, getting regular exercise, staying hydrated, and getting enough sleep are essential for maintaining good health.

    - **Avoiding Triggers**: Certain factors, such as illness, hormonal changes, or exposure to sunlight, can trigger outbreaks in some individuals. Being mindful of these triggers and taking steps to avoid them can help reduce the frequency of outbreaks.

4. **Preventing Transmission**: To reduce the risk of transmitting herpes to others, individuals should:

    - **Use Condoms**: Consistent condom use during all sexual activities can reduce the risk of transmission, even if there are no visible sores. However, condoms do not provide complete protection, as the virus can be spread from areas not covered by a condom.

- **Avoid Sexual Activity During Outbreaks**: The risk of transmitting herpes is highest during an active outbreak. It is important to avoid sexual contact when sores are present and to wait until all sores have healed before resuming sexual activity.

- **Communicate Openly**: It is crucial for individuals with genital herpes to communicate openly with their partners about their condition. Discussing the risks, preventive measures, and treatment options can help both parties make informed decisions about sexual health.

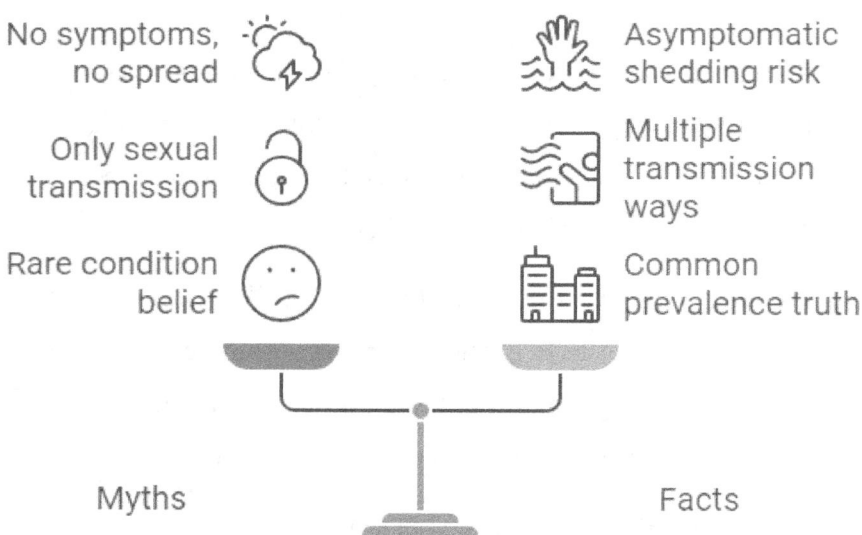

Myths vs. Facts about Genital Herpes

Conclusion

Genital herpes is a widespread and manageable condition that, with the right treatment and lifestyle adjustments, need not severely impact one's life. By debunking myths, understanding the facts, and learning how to manage outbreaks effectively, individuals with genital herpes can lead fulfilling, healthy lives. Awareness, communication, and prevention are key in reducing the stigma associated with herpes and ensuring that those affected by the condition are empowered to take control of their sexual and overall health.

Chapter 14

Gonorrhea: Symptoms, Diagnosis, and Treatment

What is Gonorrhea and How is it Transmitted?

Gonorrhea is a sexually transmitted infection (STI) caused by the bacterium *Neisseria gonorrhoeae*. This infection is one of the most common STIs worldwide and can affect both men and women. Gonorrhea can infect various mucous membranes of the body, including those of the genital tract, rectum, and throat. In rare cases, gonorrhea can also affect the eyes, joints, and bloodstream, leading to more severe complications.

Gonorrhea is primarily transmitted through sexual contact, including vaginal, anal, and oral sex. The bacteria are spread through the exchange of bodily fluids, such as semen, vaginal fluids, and rectal fluids. The infection can also be passed from an infected mother to her baby during childbirth, resulting in neonatal gonorrhea, which can lead to eye infections and, in some cases, more serious complications in newborns.

The bacterium that causes gonorrhea infects the mucosal surfaces of the reproductive tract, causing inflammation and producing the symptoms typically associated with the disease. If left untreated, gonorrhea can cause serious health problems, particularly in women, as it can lead to pelvic inflammatory disease (PID) and infertility. While gonorrhea is treatable with antibiotics, timely diagnosis and intervention are crucial to avoid long-term health issues.

Symptoms of Gonorrhea

The symptoms of gonorrhea can vary widely depending on the site of infection, and in many cases, individuals may not exhibit symptoms at all. This is particularly true for women, which makes gonorrhea challenging to detect and more likely to be transmitted unknowingly. When symptoms do occur, they tend to show up within a few days to weeks after exposure, although some people may not notice symptoms until much later. Let's explore the symptoms in both men and women.

1. **Symptoms in Women**

In women, gonorrhea often affects the cervix, urethra, and rectum. The majority of women infected with gonorrhea may not show noticeable symptoms. However, when symptoms do occur, they can include:

- **Abnormal Vaginal Discharge**: One of the most common symptoms of gonorrhea in women is an unusual discharge from the vagina, which may be yellow, green, or bloody.
- **Painful Urination**: Women infected with gonorrhea may experience a burning sensation when urinating due to the infection in the urethra.
- **Pelvic Pain**: Some women may experience pain or discomfort in the lower abdomen or pelvis, which can indicate the infection has spread to the uterus or fallopian tubes.
- **Vaginal Bleeding**: Women with gonorrhea may experience bleeding between periods or after intercourse.
- **Pain during Intercourse**: Discomfort or pain during sexual activity may occur as a result of inflammation in the cervix or reproductive organs.

If left untreated, gonorrhea in women can lead to pelvic inflammatory disease (PID), which is an infection of the reproductive organs that can cause chronic pain, infertility, and an increased risk of ectopic pregnancy.

2. **Symptoms in Men**

In men, gonorrhea tends to affect the urethra, rectum, and throat, leading to different symptoms. The most common symptoms in men include:

- **Painful Urination**: Like women, men with gonorrhea may experience a burning sensation while urinating.
- **Discharge from the Penis**: Men often notice a yellow, green, or white discharge from the tip of the penis, which can be a hallmark sign of gonorrhea.
- **Swollen or Painful Testicles**: Gonorrhea can cause pain or swelling in the testicles, which may lead to conditions such as epididymitis (inflammation of the tubes behind the testicles) if not treated promptly.
- **Sore Throat**: Men who engage in oral sex with an infected partner can contract gonorrhea in the throat, resulting in symptoms such as a sore throat, difficulty swallowing, or swollen lymph nodes.
- **Rectal Symptoms**: If the infection affects the rectum, men may experience rectal pain, itching, bleeding, or discharge, especially if they have engaged in anal sex.

Just like in women, gonorrhea can lead to complications in men, such as epididymitis, prostatitis (inflammation of the prostate), and infertility if the infection is not treated properly.

3. **Asymptomatic Gonorrhea**

One of the most concerning aspects of gonorrhea is that many individuals, particularly women, do not show any symptoms. This means that they may unknowingly spread the infection to others. Even without symptoms, untreated gonorrhea can still cause serious health complications. For example, the bacteria can spread to the upper reproductive tract in women, causing pelvic inflammatory disease (PID), or to the joints and bloodstream in both men and women.

Diagnosis of Gonorrhea

Diagnosing gonorrhea typically involves a simple test. Because the infection can affect different parts of the body, the type of test will depend on the location of the symptoms and risk factors. Common diagnostic methods include:

1. **Urine Test**: A urine test is one of the easiest ways to diagnose gonorrhea. The patient is asked to provide a urine sample, which is then tested for the presence of *Neisseria gonorrhoeae.*

2. **Swab Samples**: If the infection is suspected to be in the throat, urethra, cervix, or rectum, a healthcare provider may take a swab of the affected area. The sample is then sent to a laboratory for testing, where it is cultured or examined for the presence of the bacteria.

3. **NAAT (Nucleic Acid Amplification Test)**: This is a highly sensitive test used to detect the genetic material of the gonorrhea-causing bacteria. NAAT is one of the most accurate and common methods for diagnosing gonorrhea.

4. **Blood Test**: In rare cases, gonorrhea can spread to the bloodstream or joints. A blood test may be used to confirm the infection if there is a suspicion that the infection has reached these areas.

Early diagnosis and treatment are critical for preventing complications. Gonorrhea can be treated effectively with antibiotics, but delayed treatment can lead to more severe health issues, particularly in women.

Treatment Options for Gonorrhea

Fortunately, gonorrhea is treatable with antibiotics. The treatment usually consists of a single dose of antibiotics, though in some cases, a longer course may be required, depending on the severity of the infection. It is important for both individuals and their sexual partners to receive treatment simultaneously to prevent reinfection.

1. **Antibiotics**: The most common treatment for gonorrhea is a combination of antibiotics, usually administered as an injection and/or oral medications. The Centers for Disease Control and Prevention (CDC) currently recommends a dual therapy regimen consisting of:

    - **Ceftriaxone (Rocephin)**: A single dose of this antibiotic is administered via an injection.

    - **Azithromycin**: A single dose of this oral antibiotic is taken along with the ceftriaxone injection to combat the bacteria more effectively.

Antibiotic resistance is a growing concern, and certain strains of gonorrhea have developed resistance to commonly used antibiotics, which is why combination therapy is now the standard.

2. **Treatment for Complications**: If gonorrhea has led to complications such as pelvic inflammatory disease (PID) or epididymitis, additional treatment may be necessary, including a longer course of antibiotics or even hospitalization if the infection has spread significantly.

3. **Follow-Up Testing**: After treatment, follow-up testing may be recommended to ensure that the infection has been completely cleared,

especially for individuals who are at risk of reinfection or who had complications during their initial diagnosis.

Prevention Methods for Gonorrhea

The best way to prevent gonorrhea is to take precautions that reduce the risk of sexual transmission. Here are some effective prevention methods:

1. **Use Condoms**: Consistent and correct use of condoms during vaginal, anal, and oral sex is one of the most effective ways to prevent gonorrhea and other STIs. Condoms help reduce direct contact with infected bodily fluids, lowering the risk of transmission.

2. **Limit Sexual Partners**: Reducing the number of sexual partners can lower the risk of contracting gonorrhea. Individuals in mutually monogamous relationships, where both partners are uninfected, have a lower risk of contracting STIs.

3. **Regular STI Testing**: Regular testing is crucial, especially for individuals who have multiple sexual partners or engage in unprotected sex. Early detection of gonorrhea and other STIs can prevent complications and transmission to others.

4. **Avoid Sexual Activity During Outbreaks**: If either partner has symptoms of gonorrhea, including sores, discharge, or pain, sexual activity should be avoided until both individuals have completed treatment and received confirmation that the infection has been cleared.

5. **Communication with Sexual Partners**: Open and honest communication about STI testing, treatment, and prevention can help individuals make informed decisions about sexual health and reduce the spread of gonorrhea.

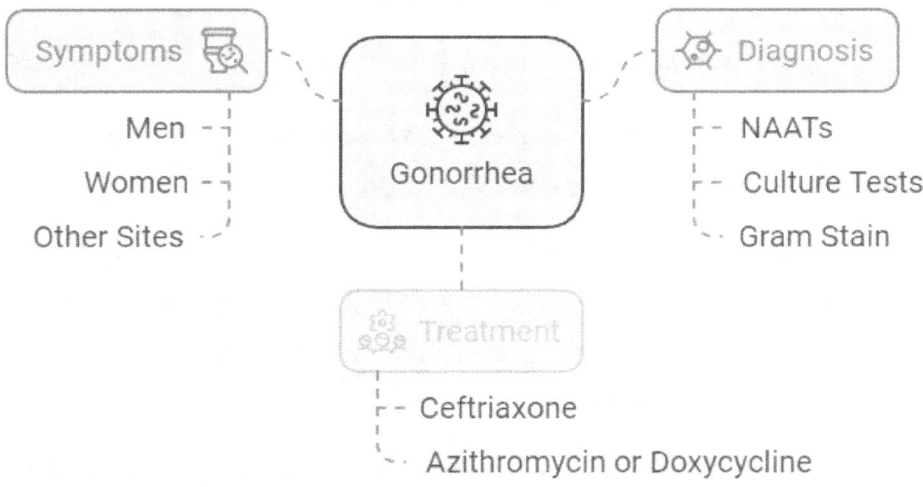

Conclusion

Gonorrhea is a highly treatable but often underdiagnosed STI that can cause significant health complications if left untreated. Early detection and treatment with antibiotics are essential for preventing serious long-term effects such as infertility and chronic pain. The symptoms of gonorrhea can be subtle, particularly in women, so regular STI testing and open communication with sexual partners are crucial to reducing the spread of this infection. By practicing safe sex, getting tested regularly, and seeking treatment promptly, individuals can protect their reproductive health and well-being from gonorrhea and its potential complications.

Chapter 15

The Psychological Impact of STIs
Coping with the Emotional and Mental Health Effects of STI Diagnoses

The diagnosis of a sexually transmitted infection (STI) can have profound psychological effects on an individual. Whether the infection is recent or chronic, the emotional and mental health impacts can be significant, affecting various aspects of life, including self-esteem, relationships, and overall well-being. Understanding the psychological toll of STIs and how to effectively cope with it is a critical component of managing one's sexual health.

Upon learning of an STI diagnosis, individuals may experience a range of emotions, including fear, shame, guilt, anger, and confusion. These emotions can stem from the perceived social stigma attached to STIs, the impact on one's health, or concerns about future fertility or complications. Additionally, some individuals may face anxiety about the implications for their relationships and worry about transmitting the infection to a partner. These emotional reactions are natural but can become overwhelming if not addressed properly.

1. **Fear and Anxiety**: One of the most common psychological responses to an STI diagnosis is fear. Fear of the unknown, fear of judgment from others, and fear of long-term health complications can all contribute to heightened levels of anxiety. In many cases, individuals may be concerned about the possibility of infertility, chronic illness, or the prospect of living with a lifelong condition.

Additionally, the fear of transmission to others—especially close partners or future partners—can lead to feelings of guilt or anxiety about how to navigate relationships moving forward. This anxiety can also manifest as hyperawareness of symptoms, excessive worry about future outbreaks, or constant concerns about whether the infection will recur.

2. **Shame and Guilt**: Social stigma surrounding STIs can lead to feelings of shame and guilt. Many individuals diagnosed with an STI may internalize the belief that they are somehow "dirty" or morally compromised, even though STIs are common and can be contracted by anyone, regardless of their sexual history or practices. This sense of shame can be exacerbated by societal attitudes that often portray people with STIs as irresponsible or promiscuous. These feelings of shame can contribute to self-blame, which may prevent the individual from seeking appropriate medical care or discussing the condition openly with partners.

Guilt may also arise if the person feels responsible for passing the infection to others, especially if they were unaware of their own infection or if the diagnosis occurs after sexual activity. The emotional weight of carrying these feelings can impair mental health, leading to issues like depression or a sense of isolation.

3. **Depression**: The mental health consequences of STI diagnoses can lead to depression in some individuals. Feelings of worthlessness, hopelessness, or sadness may arise due to the perceived long-term impact of the STI on one's life. Depression may also stem from the anxiety and stress of managing the infection or facing a future where one may need to continue dealing with the health condition. In cases where the STI leads to chronic symptoms or complications, such as infertility or painful outbreaks, depression may be further compounded by the physical burden of the disease.

Individuals with a history of depression or other mental health challenges may be at an increased risk for experiencing depressive symptoms following an

STI diagnosis. For some, the stigma and isolation they feel due to their diagnosis may be a contributing factor to the onset or worsening of depression.

4. **Anger**: Anger is another common response to an STI diagnosis. People may direct their anger toward themselves, their sexual partners, or the situation at large. This anger may stem from feelings of betrayal or frustration about how the infection was contracted, particularly if the STI was transmitted by a partner who was either unaware or untruthful about their own health status. Additionally, anger may arise from the perception of injustice, particularly if the person feels that they did not deserve the infection or did not engage in high-risk behavior.

For some individuals, anger can lead to destructive behaviors, such as avoiding necessary medical care, refusing to engage in treatment, or withdrawing from social and sexual interactions altogether. Addressing this anger is vital to avoid the negative mental health consequences that can arise from it.

5. **Identity and Body Image Issues**: An STI diagnosis can also affect one's self-perception and body image. This is particularly true if the STI causes visible symptoms, such as genital sores or warts. Many people feel embarrassed or self-conscious about how they look, especially if they believe that others may notice these physical signs. The stigma of having an STI can contribute to these negative feelings, affecting one's overall sense of attractiveness, desirability, and self-worth.

Additionally, chronic symptoms or recurrent infections may cause ongoing physical changes, which can further impact body image and sexual confidence. The fear of rejection or judgment from partners can lead to difficulty in accepting one's body or identity as a sexual being, which can result in withdrawing from intimate relationships altogether.

Relationship Communication and Stigma

The emotional and mental health effects of an STI diagnosis are often compounded by relationship dynamics. For many individuals, disclosing an STI diagnosis to a partner can be a daunting and stressful experience. Fear of rejection, judgment, or strain on the relationship can make it difficult to have open and honest conversations about sexual health.

1. **Disclosure and Fear of Rejection**: One of the most significant emotional challenges of an STI diagnosis is disclosing it to a partner. Fear of rejection is common, especially if the individual feels their partner may not understand or accept the condition. Many people worry that an STI diagnosis will lead to the breakdown of the relationship, or that their partner may end the relationship or lose trust in them.

This fear of rejection may also be linked to feelings of guilt or shame about the infection. Some individuals may worry that their partner will judge them as irresponsible or promiscuous, even though STIs can be contracted in a variety of ways. The thought of losing a relationship due to an STI diagnosis can add immense emotional pressure on the individual, making it difficult to have honest and open communication about the condition.

2. **Stigma and Social Judgment**: Beyond personal relationships, the societal stigma surrounding STIs can have a profound effect on individuals' mental health. The perception that people with STIs are somehow morally flawed or unclean can make it difficult for individuals to feel accepted or understood.

This stigma can contribute to social isolation, as individuals may feel embarrassed to share their diagnosis with friends, family, or colleagues.

The fear of judgment or discrimination may also prevent individuals from seeking treatment or medical care. This social stigma can be especially damaging for individuals who may have contracted the STI innocently, such as through a partner who was unfaithful or unaware of their own infection. When stigma is internalized, it can contribute to feelings of shame, low self-esteem, and even self-harm.

3. **Impact on Sexual Relationships**: STIs can also create significant challenges in sexual relationships. Both partners may experience fear or anxiety about the transmission of the infection, which can lead to changes in sexual practices, including abstaining from sex or using condoms consistently. For some couples, the STI diagnosis may cause strain in the relationship, as they navigate how to maintain intimacy and trust while managing the infection.

Couples may also experience tension related to the blame for the STI diagnosis. Miscommunication, mistrust, or unresolved anger between partners can lead to conflict, further complicating emotional and sexual intimacy. These challenges can be mitigated by open, honest communication, mutual understanding, and a shared commitment to managing the STI together.

Support Systems and Counseling Options

The psychological impact of an STI diagnosis is significant, but it is possible to manage and mitigate these effects through support systems and professional counseling. Seeking help from mental health professionals, as well as leaning on trusted friends, family, and support groups, can provide a vital source of comfort and guidance during this difficult time.

1. **Mental Health Counseling**: Talking to a therapist or counselor can be an invaluable resource for managing the emotional distress that comes with an STI diagnosis. Cognitive-behavioral therapy (CBT), for example, can help individuals challenge negative thought patterns, such as self-blame or feelings of worthlessness, and replace them with more positive, balanced perspectives. Therapy can also help individuals process feelings of anxiety, depression, or anger related to the diagnosis.

Couples counseling may be beneficial for partners who are navigating the impact of an STI on their relationship. A therapist can provide strategies for improving communication, rebuilding trust, and managing the emotional strain of living with an STI together.

2. **Support Groups**: Support groups, both in-person and online, can provide a sense of community for individuals dealing with the psychological effects of an STI diagnosis. These groups allow people to share their experiences, seek advice, and offer encouragement to others who are facing similar challenges. Many individuals find comfort in knowing they are not alone and that others understand the emotional toll of managing an STI.

Support groups can also be a valuable resource for learning more about the STI itself, treatment options, and coping strategies. These groups provide a space where people can openly discuss their experiences without fear of judgment, helping to reduce the stigma and shame associated with STIs.

3. **Education and Empowerment**: One of the most effective ways to cope with the psychological effects of an STI diagnosis is to become informed

about the infection. Educating oneself about the nature of the STI, how it is transmitted, and the treatment options available can help alleviate fear and uncertainty. Knowledge can empower individuals to take control of their sexual health and reduce the anxiety that often accompanies an STI diagnosis.

Additionally, sexual health education can be particularly helpful for understanding safe sex practices, the importance of regular testing, and how to prevent future infections. When individuals feel empowered with knowledge, they are better equipped to manage their health and relationships without the added burden of fear or shame.

Psychological Impact of STIs

- Emotional Responses
  - Anxiety and Fear
  - Depression
  - Secrecy
  - Societal Judgment
  - Stigma
- Relationship Dynamics
  - Transmission Anxiety
  - Communication Barriers
  - Support Groups
  - Counseling
  - Mental Health Support

Psychological Impact of STIs

Conclusion

The psychological impact of an STI diagnosis is profound and multifaceted, affecting an individual's mental health, relationships, and overall quality of life. Coping with the emotional consequences of the diagnosis—such as fear, shame, depression, and anxiety—requires time, support, and understanding. Open communication with partners, seeking professional counseling, and connecting with support groups are all valuable tools for managing the emotional impact of an STI. Reducing stigma through education, empathy, and advocacy is also crucial to improving mental health outcomes for individuals with STIs. With the right resources and coping strategies, individuals can effectively navigate the psychological challenges of an STI diagnosis and move toward a healthier, more empowered future.

Chapter 16

Prevention and Safe Practices: A Guide to Protecting Reproductive Health

Introduction to Reproductive Health Protection

Maintaining optimal reproductive health involves more than just addressing existing conditions. Prevention is an essential aspect of sexual and reproductive health that empowers individuals to safeguard their well-being and avoid the onset of sexually transmitted infections (STIs) and other reproductive health issues. By adopting safe sex practices, utilizing contraception, staying up to date with vaccinations, and committing to regular STI screenings, individuals can reduce their risk of complications and maintain better overall reproductive health.

This chapter provides a comprehensive guide to protecting reproductive health by exploring safe sex practices, contraception options, vaccination strategies, and the importance of regular STI screening. It is essential to not only prioritize prevention to avoid harm but also to educate oneself on the choices available to reduce risks and ensure long-term sexual health.

Safe Sex Practices: The Foundation of Protection

Safe sex refers to practices that reduce the likelihood of sexually transmitted infections (STIs) and unintended pregnancies. By understanding and implementing safe sex practices, individuals take proactive steps to protect their reproductive health and that of their partners.

1. **Condom Use**: One of the most widely recommended forms of protection during sexual activity is the use of condoms. Both male and female condoms serve as effective barriers against the transmission of STIs, including HIV, herpes, gonorrhea, chlamydia, and syphilis. Male condoms are worn on the

penis, while female condoms are worn inside the vagina, creating a physical barrier to prevent bodily fluids from mixing.

Consistent and correct use of condoms during vaginal, anal, and oral sex significantly reduces the risk of STI transmission. However, it is important to note that while condoms offer excellent protection, they are not 100% effective in preventing all STIs. This is especially true for infections that spread through skin-to-skin contact, such as genital herpes or human papillomavirus (HPV). Nonetheless, condoms remain one of the best preventive measures available for reducing STI risks.

2. **Dental Dams**: For individuals engaging in oral sex, dental dams offer a protective barrier between the mouth and the genital area, preventing the exchange of bodily fluids and reducing the transmission of STIs. Dental dams, which are thin, flexible sheets of latex or polyurethane, are used in oral-vaginal and oral-anal sex. Just as with condoms, using dental dams consistently helps minimize the risk of infection and ensures safer sexual practices. While they are not as widely used as condoms, dental dams are an important tool in protecting reproductive health.

3. **Mutual Monogamy**: One of the safest sexual practices for preventing STIs is engaging in a mutually monogamous relationship in which both partners are tested for STIs and remain exclusive to one another. By committing to sexual exclusivity and being open about sexual health, couples can reduce the likelihood of STI transmission. It is essential that both partners are tested before discontinuing other protective measures like condom use. In such relationships, the risk of STI exposure is minimized, but regular health check-ups are still important.

4. **Communication and Consent**: Effective communication about sexual health and consent is critical to maintaining safe practices. Having an open dialogue with a partner about STIs, condom use, and contraception is vital to ensure both individuals are informed and on the same page. Clear communication can prevent misunderstandings, help in making informed decisions, and create a sense of shared responsibility for both partners' health and well-being. Consent and communication also help to avoid coercive or non-consensual situations, promoting healthier, safer sexual encounters.

5. **Limiting the Number of Sexual Partners**: Reducing the number of sexual partners can help minimize the exposure to potential STIs. While having multiple sexual partners increases the risk of infection, engaging in fewer sexual encounters with trusted partners reduces overall exposure. It is also important to ensure that all partners are tested for STIs and that safe sex practices are used consistently, regardless of the number of partners.

Contraception: Preventing Unintended Pregnancies

In addition to preventing the transmission of STIs, contraception plays a crucial role in preventing unintended pregnancies. By using birth control methods, individuals and couples can make informed decisions about their reproductive health and timing of pregnancy. Contraception methods range from hormonal to barrier methods and long-term solutions.

1. **Barrier Methods**: Barrier methods such as condoms, diaphragms, and cervical caps physically block sperm from reaching the egg, preventing pregnancy. Male and female condoms, as discussed earlier, are also effective at preventing both pregnancy and the transmission of STIs. Diaphragms and cervical caps are inserted into the vagina before intercourse to cover the

cervix and block sperm from entering the uterus. When used correctly, these methods are effective, though they may be less reliable than hormonal or permanent contraceptive options.

2. **Hormonal Contraception**: Hormonal birth control methods, including birth control pills, patches, injections, and intrauterine devices (IUDs), work by regulating the female reproductive system to prevent ovulation (the release of an egg), making fertilization impossible. The pill and the patch require consistent use and regular attention, while the IUD provides long-term, low-maintenance protection, as it is inserted by a healthcare provider and can last for several years.

In addition to preventing pregnancy, some hormonal methods can also offer benefits such as regulating menstrual cycles, reducing menstrual cramps, and improving conditions like acne or endometriosis. However, they do not protect against STIs, so they are best used in combination with condoms for comprehensive sexual health protection.

3. **Sterilization**: For individuals or couples who are certain they do not want to have children, permanent sterilization options such as tubal ligation (for women) or vasectomy (for men) provide effective, permanent contraception. These methods are highly reliable and require careful consideration before choosing, as they are not reversible. While sterilization does not protect against STIs, it is an option for those who have completed their families or have decided not to have children.

4. **Natural Family Planning**: Natural family planning (NFP), or fertility awareness, involves tracking a woman's menstrual cycle and avoiding sex during the most fertile times to prevent pregnancy. While this method relies

on careful attention to the body's natural signals (such as temperature and cervical mucus), it is less reliable than other methods of contraception. NFP does not provide protection against STIs and may be less effective for individuals with irregular menstrual cycles.

5. **Emergency Contraception**: In cases where unprotected sex occurs or contraception fails, emergency contraception (EC) pills, also known as the "morning-after pill," can be taken to prevent pregnancy. These pills contain hormones that delay ovulation, preventing fertilization. Emergency contraception is not an abortion pill, and it is most effective when taken within 72 hours of unprotected intercourse, though it can work up to five days in some cases. It is important to note that emergency contraception does not protect against STIs.

Vaccination Options: Preventive Measures for Reproductive Health

Vaccination plays an important role in preventing certain types of STIs, especially those that can lead to long-term health complications like cancer. Vaccines can protect against the most common infections that affect reproductive health, offering individuals an opportunity to reduce their risk.

1. **Human Papillomavirus (HPV) Vaccine**: HPV is one of the most common STIs worldwide, with certain strains causing genital warts and others linked to cancers such as cervical, anal, and throat cancer. The HPV vaccine is a highly effective preventive measure that protects against the most dangerous strains of the virus, such as HPV-16 and HPV-18. Administered in a series of doses, the vaccine is recommended for preteens, but it can also be given to individuals up to the age of 26, and in some cases, up to 45.

Vaccination significantly reduces the risk of developing HPV-related cancers and genital warts. While the vaccine does not protect against all types of HPV, it is still one of the most effective ways to prevent serious reproductive health issues. It is most effective when given before any sexual activity, as it works best in those who have not yet been exposed to the virus.

2. **Hepatitis B Vaccine**: Hepatitis B is a viral infection that affects the liver and is transmitted through bodily fluids, including blood and semen. It can be passed through sexual contact, sharing needles, and from mother to child during childbirth. Chronic hepatitis B infection can lead to liver disease and cancer. The hepatitis B vaccine is effective in preventing this infection and is typically given as a series of three shots. Vaccination is recommended for all infants, but adults who are at higher risk—such as those who have multiple sexual partners or engage in intravenous drug use—should also consider getting vaccinated.

Promoting Regular STI Screening

Regular STI screening is a cornerstone of reproductive health and prevention. Testing for STIs allows individuals to catch infections early, even when symptoms are not present, and reduce the risk of complications. Many STIs can be asymptomatic for long periods, making testing essential for sexually active individuals.

1. **Frequency of Testing**: The Centers for Disease Control and Prevention (CDC) recommends routine STI screenings for sexually active individuals, particularly those with multiple partners or unprotected sex. Women under 25 should be tested for chlamydia and gonorrhea every year, while

individuals who engage in high-risk behaviors, such as having unprotected sex or sharing needles, should be tested for a wider range of STIs.

2. **Comprehensive Testing**: Comprehensive STI testing typically includes screenings for a range of infections, such as HIV, syphilis, herpes, gonorrhea, and chlamydia. Some clinics also offer testing for other STIs like trichomoniasis, hepatitis, and HPV. Testing can be done through urine samples, blood tests, or swabs of the genital area, depending on the infection being tested for.

3. **Partner Testing**: It is important for sexual partners to get tested together, particularly if one partner has tested positive for an STI. Partner testing helps to ensure both individuals are informed and can take necessary precautions to avoid reinfection or transmission.

4. **Confidentiality and Access to Care**: STI screenings are confidential, and individuals should feel empowered to seek testing without fear of judgment or discrimination. Many public health clinics, sexual health centers, and primary care providers offer free or low-cost STI testing. Early diagnosis and treatment can prevent serious health complications and ensure that individuals remain informed about their sexual health.

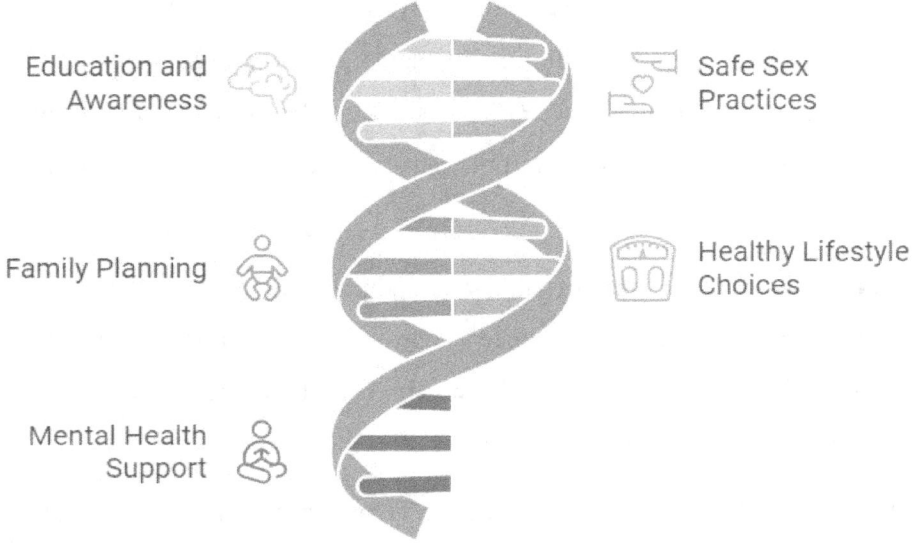

Conclusion

Prevention is the foundation of reproductive health, and adopting safe sex practices, using contraception, staying up to date on vaccinations, and committing to regular STI screenings are essential for protecting oneself and one's partners from STIs and other reproductive health issues. By prioritizing these preventive measures, individuals can enjoy healthier, safer sexual experiences and reduce their risk of long-term complications. Empowering oneself with knowledge and taking proactive steps to protect reproductive health ensures a future of well-being and informed decision-making in sexual and reproductive matters.

Chapter 17

Holistic Health Approaches to Reproductive Wellness

Introduction to Holistic Health for Reproductive Wellness

Reproductive health is often viewed through a medical lens, focusing on diagnosis, treatment, and surgery when necessary. However, an integrative or holistic approach to reproductive wellness takes into account the interconnectedness of mind, body, and spirit. This approach emphasizes not just symptom management but also the prevention of reproductive health issues by addressing the underlying factors that influence overall well-being. Holistic health strategies—such as proper nutrition, regular exercise, stress management, and the use of natural remedies—can support the body's natural ability to heal and maintain a healthy reproductive system.

This chapter explores the importance of adopting a holistic perspective in caring for reproductive health. It highlights the ways in which nutrition, physical activity, stress management, and complementary therapies can enhance reproductive wellness, improve fertility, and address a wide range of reproductive concerns. By integrating these practices into daily life, individuals can support their reproductive systems in a balanced, sustainable way, reducing the risk of conditions such as infertility, menstrual irregularities, and even more serious reproductive health challenges.

Nutrition: Fueling the Reproductive System

Nutrition plays a crucial role in maintaining reproductive health. A balanced, nutrient-rich diet can have a profound impact on hormonal balance, fertility, and overall reproductive function. Many reproductive health issues—such as polycystic ovary syndrome (PCOS), endometriosis, and male infertility—can be influenced by poor dietary habits or nutrient deficiencies. Proper nutrition helps to support healthy hormone production, regulate menstrual cycles, and increase the likelihood of conception for both men and women.

1. **Key Nutrients for Reproductive Health**: Several key vitamins and minerals are critical for maintaining reproductive health, and deficiencies in these nutrients can impair fertility. These nutrients include:

    - **Folic Acid**: Essential for women who are planning to conceive, folic acid helps to reduce the risk of neural tube defects and supports the development of a healthy pregnancy. It also plays a role in regulating ovulation and improving fertility.

    - **Vitamin D**: Studies have shown that adequate levels of vitamin D are linked to improved fertility outcomes in both men and women. Vitamin D plays a role in regulating hormone levels and supporting a healthy menstrual cycle. For men, it may also contribute to higher testosterone levels and sperm quality.

    - **Zinc**: Zinc is essential for both male and female reproductive health. In women, it helps to regulate hormone production, while in men, it supports sperm production and motility. Zinc deficiency has been linked to reduced fertility in both genders.

    - **Omega-3 Fatty Acids**: Omega-3 fatty acids, found in fatty fish such as salmon, flax seeds, and walnuts, are anti-inflammatory and support healthy ovulation and sperm quality. They are particularly important for managing conditions like PCOS and endometriosis, which can lead to fertility issues.

- **Antioxidants**: Vitamins A, C, and E, as well as selenium, are powerful antioxidants that help to protect the reproductive organs from oxidative stress. This is especially important for women with conditions like endometriosis or fibroids, as oxidative damage can exacerbate these conditions. For men, antioxidants can help to protect sperm from DNA damage and improve overall fertility.

2. **Foods to Include in a Reproductive Health Diet**: A balanced, fertility-friendly diet includes whole, nutrient-dense foods such as:
    - Leafy greens (spinach, kale)
    - Whole grains (brown rice, quinoa, oats)
    - Berries and citrus fruits (rich in antioxidants)
    - Lean proteins (chicken, turkey, tofu)
    - Healthy fats (avocados, olive oil, nuts)
    - Fish high in omega-3s (salmon, sardines)
    - Legumes (lentils, chickpeas, beans)
    - Dairy or calcium-rich alternatives (for hormone balance)

3. **Foods to Avoid**: While some foods support reproductive health, others can negatively impact fertility and hormonal balance. Highly processed foods, excessive caffeine, sugar, trans fats, and alcohol can contribute to inflammation, insulin resistance, and hormonal imbalances that may hinder reproductive health. Reducing the intake of these foods can help to support healthy hormone levels and improve fertility outcomes.

Exercise: Enhancing Fertility through Physical Activity

Physical activity has a significant impact on reproductive health, influencing hormone levels, metabolism, and overall well-being. Regular exercise promotes a healthy body weight, reduces stress, and improves blood circulation to the reproductive organs, all of which contribute to a balanced reproductive system. However, the intensity and type of exercise matter, as both over-exercising and under-exercising can negatively affect fertility.

1. **Exercise and Female Reproductive Health**: For women, regular moderate exercise has been shown to improve menstrual regularity and support healthy ovulation. Exercise also helps manage body weight, which is important for women with conditions such as PCOS, where obesity can exacerbate hormonal imbalances. Additionally, regular exercise promotes better circulation to the reproductive organs, which can support the overall health of the ovaries, uterus, and fallopian tubes.

    - **Recommended Activities**: Aerobic exercises such as walking, cycling, swimming, and low-impact activities like yoga or Pilates can help maintain a healthy weight, improve mood, and reduce stress. Strength training exercises are also beneficial for building muscle mass and enhancing metabolic function.

2. **Exercise and Male Reproductive Health**: For men, regular physical activity improves sperm quality, motility, and overall reproductive health. Exercise helps maintain a healthy body weight, improve cardiovascular health, and reduce inflammation, which can positively influence sperm production and function. Like women, men should avoid excessive exercise, which can lead to hormonal imbalances and a decline in sperm quality.

- **Recommended Activities**: Moderate-intensity exercises such as jogging, swimming, cycling, and resistance training can help maintain sperm health. Exercise that targets the core and pelvic floor muscles can also improve sexual function and support reproductive health.

3. **Balancing Exercise**: While exercise is crucial for reproductive health, too much of it can have adverse effects. Over-exercising, especially in women, can lead to irregular menstrual cycles, hormonal imbalances, and even fertility problems. Intense physical activity, combined with inadequate nutrition, can lead to a condition called hypothalamic amenorrhea, where the menstrual cycle stops due to low body fat and stress. It's important to find a balance and avoid extreme forms of exercise, especially if you are trying to conceive.

Stress Management: Reducing the Impact on Fertility

Chronic stress is one of the most overlooked factors influencing reproductive health. High levels of stress can disrupt hormonal balance, impair ovulation, and reduce fertility in both men and women. In women, stress can affect the production of hormones like cortisol, which can interfere with the menstrual cycle and impact ovulation. In men, stress can affect testosterone levels and sperm quality. Therefore, managing stress is a key component of maintaining optimal reproductive health.

1. **The Role of Cortisol in Fertility**: Cortisol is the body's primary stress hormone, and prolonged elevated levels can disrupt the normal function of the hypothalamus, pituitary gland, and ovaries or testes. This disruption can lead to irregular periods, ovulation problems, or reduced sperm count.

Additionally, stress affects the immune system, which can worsen conditions like endometriosis or PCOS.

2. **Stress-Reducing Techniques**: Implementing regular stress-management practices can help restore hormonal balance and support fertility. Some effective techniques include:

    - **Mindfulness and Meditation**: Practices like mindfulness, meditation, and deep breathing can help activate the parasympathetic nervous system, which counteracts the stress response and promotes relaxation. These practices can be especially beneficial for women with PCOS or women undergoing fertility treatments, as they help reduce anxiety and restore balance to the hormonal system.

    - **Yoga and Tai Chi**: These ancient practices combine physical movement with breathwork, helping to release tension, increase flexibility, and improve circulation. Yoga, in particular, has been shown to reduce cortisol levels and improve reproductive health by promoting relaxation and hormone regulation.

    - **Journaling and Cognitive Behavioral Therapy (CBT)**: Journaling can be a powerful tool for expressing emotions and releasing pent-up stress. CBT is a form of therapy that helps individuals identify and challenge negative thought patterns that contribute to anxiety and stress.

3. **Sleep and Rest**: Adequate rest is vital for reproductive health. Sleep deprivation, often linked to high stress, can lead to hormonal imbalances and interfere with ovulation. Ensuring a regular sleep schedule of 7-9 hours per night is essential for reducing stress and promoting reproductive wellness.

Natural Remedies for Reproductive Health

In addition to lifestyle changes such as nutrition, exercise, and stress management, several natural remedies may support reproductive health. While these remedies should not replace medical treatment, they can be used as complementary strategies to promote balance and healing.

1. **Herbal Supplements**: Certain herbs have been shown to support reproductive health by balancing hormones and improving fertility. Some popular herbs for women include:

    - **Maca Root**: Known for its ability to balance hormones and improve energy levels, maca root is commonly used to support fertility and regulate menstrual cycles.
    - **Chaste Tree Berry (Vitex)**: This herb is often used to treat menstrual irregularities and support ovulation. It works by regulating the pituitary gland and helping to balance estrogen and progesterone levels.
    - **Red Clover**: Rich in phytoestrogens, red clover can help balance estrogen levels and support overall reproductive health in women.

    For men, herbs such as **ashwagandha**, which is believed to support sperm production and testosterone levels, and **Tribulus Terrestris**, which may improve libido and reproductive health, have shown promise.

2. **Acupuncture**: Acupuncture is a form of Traditional Chinese Medicine (TCM) that involves inserting fine needles into specific points on the body to stimulate energy flow. It has been used to treat infertility by improving

blood flow to the reproductive organs, balancing hormones, and reducing stress.

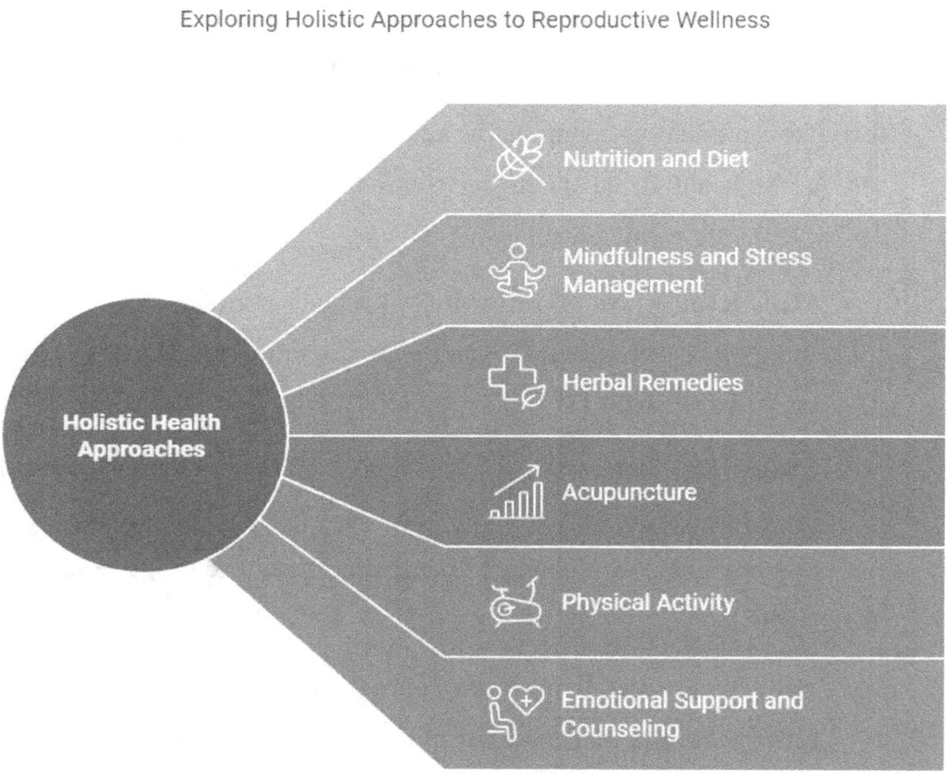

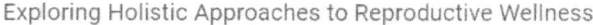

Exploring Holistic Approaches to Reproductive Wellness

Conclusion

A holistic approach to reproductive health emphasizes the importance of balancing physical, emotional, and lifestyle factors to optimize fertility and reproductive wellness. By focusing on nutrition, exercise, stress management, and natural remedies, individuals can create a supportive environment for their reproductive system, improve their chances of conception, and address a variety of reproductive health concerns. Integrating these strategies into daily life can not only help prevent reproductive issues but also enhance overall health and well-being. By nurturing both body and mind, we can foster a deeper connection to our reproductive health and ensure lasting wellness.

Chapter 18

The Role of Modern Medicine in Reproductive Health

Introduction: The Intersection of Tradition and Innovation

Reproductive health has undergone dramatic changes in the last few decades, thanks to rapid advancements in modern medicine. From assisted reproductive technologies (ART) to minimally invasive surgical techniques, modern medicine offers an array of treatments that have significantly improved the lives of individuals and couples facing reproductive challenges. These innovations have made it possible for many to experience parenthood, overcome infertility, and address a range of reproductive health issues with higher success rates than ever before. However, while these technologies and medical interventions are transformative, their long-term impact on health and their integration with traditional and holistic approaches are areas of increasing interest and importance.

This chapter delves into the advances in reproductive health technology, how modern medical interventions have shaped reproductive outcomes, and the potential of combining modern medicine with traditional practices to optimize reproductive health. Understanding these components can empower individuals to make informed decisions regarding their reproductive health and ensure that both short-term and long-term outcomes are carefully considered.

Advances in Reproductive Health Technology

In recent years, there has been a revolutionary shift in the field of reproductive medicine. Technologies once thought to be unattainable are now commonplace in fertility clinics and reproductive health centers around the world. Assisted reproductive technologies (ART) are among the most significant advancements, allowing individuals and couples to overcome infertility caused by a range of factors, including age, medical conditions, and unexplained infertility.

1. **In Vitro Fertilization (IVF)**: IVF has revolutionized the treatment of infertility by allowing eggs to be fertilized outside of the body and then implanted into the uterus. IVF has helped countless couples conceive, particularly those with conditions such as fallopian tube blockages, endometriosis, male infertility, or unexplained infertility. Over the years, IVF techniques have improved, with advancements in embryo freezing, genetic screening of embryos (PGT), and the use of egg or sperm donors.

    - **Embryo Cryopreservation**: One of the most significant breakthroughs in IVF is the ability to freeze embryos for future use. This process, known as cryopreservation, allows women to delay childbearing while preserving their fertility. It is especially beneficial for those undergoing cancer treatments or for women who want to delay pregnancy until later in life. The ability to store viable embryos provides women with options that were previously unavailable.

    - **Genetic Testing and Screening**: With the rise of genetic screening, doctors can now test embryos for genetic abnormalities before implantation, a process known as preimplantation genetic testing (PGT). PGT allows for the selection of embryos with the highest likelihood of success, reducing the risk of genetic disorders and improving the overall success rates of IVF.

2. **Egg Freezing**: Egg freezing has become a popular option for women who want to preserve their fertility for future use. This process involves stimulating the ovaries to produce multiple eggs, which are then harvested,

frozen, and stored until the woman is ready to conceive. Egg freezing has been especially beneficial for women with medical conditions, such as cancer, that may affect their fertility, as well as women who are delaying childbearing due to career or personal reasons.

3. **Fertility Preservation for Men**: Just as women have the option to freeze eggs, men can also preserve their fertility through sperm freezing. Men who are undergoing cancer treatments or who are at risk of infertility due to age or other medical conditions can freeze sperm for future use. This option has provided many men with the opportunity to have biological children after undergoing treatments that may impact their reproductive health.

4. **Artificial Insemination (IUI)**: Intrauterine insemination (IUI) is a less invasive alternative to IVF that is often used in cases of mild male infertility or unexplained infertility. It involves the direct placement of sperm into the uterus during ovulation to increase the chances of fertilization. IUI has proven to be an effective solution for many couples and is often used as a first-line treatment before moving to more advanced reproductive technologies.

5. **Fertility Drugs**: Medications that stimulate ovulation have become a cornerstone in fertility treatments. Drugs such as Clomiphene citrate (Clomid) and gonadotropins are commonly prescribed to women who have difficulty ovulating. These drugs work by stimulating the ovaries to produce more eggs, increasing the chances of conception. For men, medications such as human chorionic gonadotropin (hCG) may be used to increase sperm production in cases of low sperm count or poor sperm motility.

Medical Interventions and Their Impact on Long-Term Health

While modern reproductive medicine has made great strides in helping individuals achieve their reproductive goals, it is essential to consider the long-term effects of some interventions. The advances in ART and fertility treatments have made it easier for individuals to conceive, but as with any medical treatment, it is important to understand the potential risks and outcomes.

1. **Long-Term Health Effects of IVF**: One of the most discussed concerns regarding ART is the long-term health implications of IVF. Research has shown that IVF pregnancies may carry a slightly higher risk of complications, such as preterm birth, low birth weight, and multiple pregnancies (twins or triplets). Multiple pregnancies, while sometimes desired, come with increased risks for both the mother and the babies, including preterm labor, gestational diabetes, and high blood pressure.

    - **Genetic Concerns**: Advances in genetic testing have reduced the risk of genetic disorders in embryos, but it is still important to recognize that ART does not eliminate the possibility of birth defects or developmental issues. Additionally, IVF has been associated with an increased risk of imprinting disorders, such as Beckwith-Wiedemann syndrome, which affects the growth and development of infants.

    - **Emotional and Psychological Impact**: The emotional impact of undergoing ART can be significant. Infertility treatments can be emotionally and financially draining, and the failure of IVF cycles may lead to stress, anxiety, and depression. Many individuals undergoing fertility treatments also experience a sense of loss or grief if they are unable to conceive. It is important for healthcare providers to offer counseling and emotional support to patients as they navigate the complexities of ART.

2. **Effects of Fertility Medications**: Fertility drugs, while beneficial for many women, come with their own set of potential risks. Overuse of medications like Clomid can result in ovarian hyperstimulation syndrome (OHSS), a condition where the ovaries become swollen and painful. In rare cases, fertility medications can increase the risk of ovarian cancer, although this risk is still being studied. Fertility medications may also increase the likelihood of multiple pregnancies, which can carry risks for both mother and child.

3. **Surgical Interventions**: For conditions like endometriosis, fibroids, or blocked fallopian tubes, surgery may be required. While these procedures can improve fertility, they come with risks such as scarring, infection, or complications during recovery. Additionally, some women may face long-term effects such as changes in menstrual cycles or pelvic adhesions after surgery.

Combining Traditional and Modern Medical Practices

While modern medicine offers remarkable advancements in reproductive health, many individuals seek a more holistic approach to their care. Integrating traditional and complementary medical practices with modern reproductive technologies can provide a comprehensive approach to reproductive health. This integrative approach combines the best of both worlds—cutting-edge medical treatments and time-tested natural remedies.

1. **Acupuncture and IVF**: Acupuncture, an ancient Chinese medicine practice, has been shown to improve the success rates of IVF by promoting blood flow to the uterus and ovaries, reducing stress, and balancing hormones. Many fertility clinics now offer acupuncture as a complementary treatment

to IVF, with promising results in increasing implantation rates and reducing the risk of miscarriage.

2. **Herbal Medicine**: Herbs such as red clover, chaste tree berry (Vitex), and maca root are commonly used to support fertility in both men and women. These herbs can help regulate hormonal balance, improve ovulation, and support sperm quality. When used in conjunction with medical treatments, herbal supplements can enhance reproductive health and provide additional support to individuals undergoing fertility treatments.

3. **Nutrition and Lifestyle**: A healthy diet, regular exercise, and stress management are essential components of reproductive wellness. Many individuals who undergo ART or other medical treatments may benefit from nutritional counseling to optimize their health and improve fertility outcomes. Diets rich in antioxidants, healthy fats, and essential nutrients can improve sperm and egg quality, while exercise and stress management help reduce the negative effects of chronic stress on fertility.

4. **Mind-Body Connection**: Practices such as yoga and meditation can be incredibly beneficial for individuals dealing with fertility challenges. The mind-body connection plays a significant role in reproductive health, and managing stress through relaxation techniques can have a profound impact on hormonal regulation and fertility. Mindfulness practices also support emotional well-being, which is crucial when navigating the often-challenging emotional journey of infertility treatment.

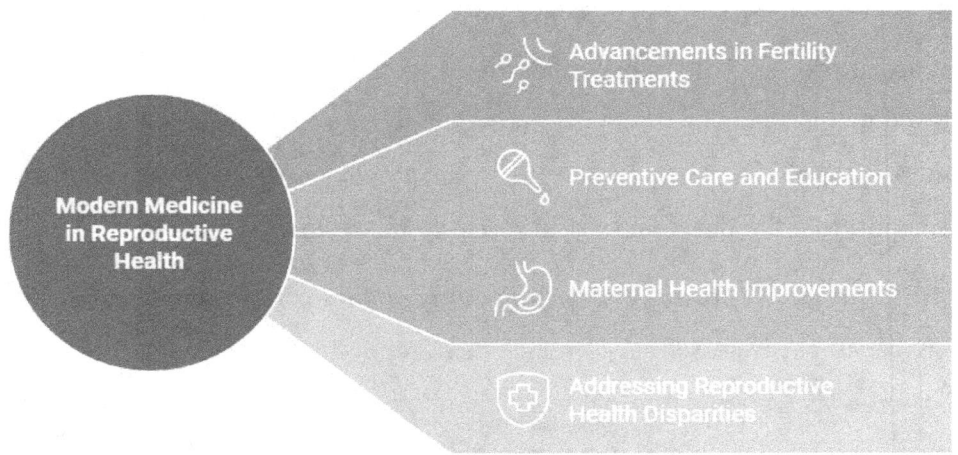

Conclusion

Modern medicine has made incredible strides in reproductive health, offering cutting-edge technologies and treatments that have helped millions of individuals and couples overcome challenges related to infertility, reproductive health disorders, and family-building. However, it is essential to take a holistic approach that combines the best of both modern and traditional medicine. By integrating advanced medical treatments with complementary therapies, individuals can optimize their reproductive health and improve their chances of success, whether they are seeking to conceive or simply maintain overall reproductive wellness.

Ultimately, the future of reproductive health lies in a balanced and integrated approach that considers the physical, emotional, and psychological aspects of the individual. With the right knowledge, support, and a holistic approach to care, individuals can achieve their reproductive goals and enjoy healthy, fulfilling lives.

Chapter 19

Lifestyle Choices and Reproductive Health

Introduction: The Connection Between Lifestyle and Reproductive Health

Reproductive health is a multifaceted aspect of well-being, influenced by various physical, environmental, and social factors. Among these, lifestyle choices play a pivotal role in determining an individual's reproductive health outcomes. While factors like genetics and age are often seen as the primary contributors to fertility and sexual health, lifestyle behaviors, such as smoking, alcohol consumption, drug use, diet, and exercise, can have profound effects on reproductive function. Understanding how these factors influence fertility and sexual health is essential for making informed decisions about one's health and well-being.

This chapter explores the relationship between lifestyle choices and reproductive health, delving into the impact of smoking, alcohol, and drug use on fertility, the ways in which weight and fitness levels affect reproductive outcomes, and the significant role that mental health plays in reproductive health. By recognizing the influence of lifestyle factors, individuals can make positive changes that improve both their immediate and long-term reproductive health outcomes.

Impact of Smoking, Alcohol, and Drug Use on Fertility and Sexual Health

1. **Smoking and Fertility**: Smoking is one of the most detrimental lifestyle choices for both men and women in relation to reproductive health. The harmful chemicals in tobacco smoke, such as nicotine and carbon monoxide,

can directly impact fertility by damaging reproductive organs, altering hormone levels, and reducing the quality of eggs and sperm.

- **In Women**: Smoking accelerates the depletion of a woman's eggs, leading to earlier menopause and a diminished ovarian reserve. It has been linked to decreased fertility rates and an increased risk of miscarriage. Additionally, smoking can cause tubal damage, which may impair the movement of eggs and sperm, increasing the risk of ectopic pregnancies. Smokers may also experience more difficulty with assisted reproduction techniques like IVF, with lower success rates compared to non-smokers.

- **In Men**: In men, smoking can negatively affect sperm quality, leading to a lower sperm count, reduced motility (movement), and abnormal sperm shape. Studies have shown that smoking can also reduce testosterone levels and impair erectile function, making it harder to conceive. Moreover, the toxins in cigarettes can cause genetic damage to sperm, increasing the likelihood of birth defects.

2. **Alcohol and Fertility**: While moderate alcohol consumption might seem harmless, excessive drinking can have serious consequences for reproductive health. Alcohol can affect both male and female fertility, impacting hormone production, ovulation, and sperm production.

    - **In Women**: Heavy alcohol consumption can disrupt menstrual cycles, leading to irregular or absent periods. It may also interfere with ovulation, making it difficult for women to conceive. Chronic alcohol use can result in liver damage, which affects estrogen metabolism, and may cause changes in hormone levels that reduce fertility. Women who drink excessively may also face an increased risk of miscarriage, preterm birth, and developmental issues in the baby.

- **In Men**: In men, heavy alcohol use can lead to hormonal imbalances, reducing testosterone levels and impairing sperm production. Alcohol has also been linked to erectile dysfunction, which may make it more difficult to engage in sexual activity. Long-term heavy drinking can lead to liver disease and other health complications that indirectly affect reproductive function.

- **Fetal Alcohol Syndrome (FAS)**: When pregnant women drink alcohol, they risk passing harmful substances to the fetus. Fetal alcohol syndrome can result in lifelong developmental and cognitive issues for the child. This underscores the importance of avoiding alcohol consumption during pregnancy and even while trying to conceive.

3. **Drug Use and Fertility**: Both prescription and recreational drug use can interfere with fertility, often by disrupting the delicate balance of hormones required for reproduction.

    - **Prescription Medications**: Some prescription medications, such as certain antidepressants, corticosteroids, and chemotherapy drugs, can affect fertility. For example, chemotherapy drugs can damage reproductive organs, impair sperm production, and reduce ovarian function. It is essential to consult with healthcare providers when taking any medication, particularly when planning to conceive, to evaluate potential effects on fertility.

- **Recreational Drugs**: Recreational drugs, such as marijuana, cocaine, and heroin, are known to have significant negative effects on reproductive health. Marijuana, while sometimes used for medical purposes, can decrease sperm motility and count in men, and may also affect ovulation in women. Cocaine use can cause reduced blood flow to the reproductive organs, leading to poor sperm quality and irregular menstrual cycles in women. Heroin can disrupt hormone production and fertility in both men and women, and long-term use can lead to infertility.
- **Managing Substance Use**: Those struggling with substance abuse are encouraged to seek professional help. Addressing these issues can improve overall health and enhance fertility. Many rehabilitation centers now offer specialized support for individuals seeking to improve their reproductive health while managing addiction.

How Weight and Fitness Levels Affect Reproductive Outcomes

1. **The Role of Healthy Weight in Fertility**: Body weight is another critical factor influencing reproductive health. Both underweight and overweight individuals may experience fertility issues due to hormonal imbalances, irregular cycles, and reduced sperm quality.
   - **Underweight**: Women who are significantly underweight may have irregular menstrual cycles or even stop menstruating altogether (amenorrhea), which can make conception more difficult. Low body fat levels can interfere with the production of estrogen, a hormone crucial for ovulation. Women with low body weight may also face a higher risk of miscarriage and preterm labor. In men, being

underweight can lead to reduced testosterone levels, lower sperm production, and poor sperm quality.

- **Overweight and Obesity**: On the other hand, being overweight or obese can also impair fertility. In women, excess fat tissue can lead to hormonal imbalances, particularly with estrogen and insulin, which can disrupt ovulation. Conditions like polycystic ovary syndrome (PCOS) are more common in women who are overweight, which can further complicate fertility. Obesity can also increase the risk of complications during pregnancy, such as gestational diabetes, high blood pressure, and preeclampsia.

- **In Men**: Obesity can reduce sperm count and motility in men, possibly due to changes in hormone levels and increased scrotal temperature. Additionally, overweight men are more likely to experience erectile dysfunction and other sexual health issues, which can impair their ability to conceive.

- **Achieving a Healthy Weight**: Maintaining a balanced, nutritious diet, engaging in regular physical activity, and striving for a healthy weight can significantly enhance fertility. For both men and women, staying within a healthy weight range improves hormonal balance and supports reproductive function. Consulting with a healthcare provider or nutritionist can be beneficial when trying to achieve an optimal weight for reproductive health.

2. **Fitness and Exercise**: Physical activity plays a crucial role in overall reproductive health. Regular exercise can help manage body weight, improve circulation to the reproductive organs, and boost hormone

production. However, the type and intensity of exercise are essential factors to consider.

- **Moderate Exercise**: Engaging in moderate exercise, such as walking, swimming, or cycling, can improve reproductive health by reducing stress, enhancing blood flow, and maintaining a healthy weight. For women, exercise helps regulate the menstrual cycle, improve insulin sensitivity, and reduce the symptoms of PCOS. For men, regular physical activity can improve sperm quality, hormone levels, and sexual function.

- **Excessive Exercise**: While moderate exercise is beneficial, excessive exercise or overtraining can have the opposite effect on fertility. Intense physical activity, especially when coupled with low body fat, can lead to hormonal disruptions, irregular menstrual cycles, and reduced sperm production. Women who engage in extreme sports or exercise routines may experience delayed or absent periods, and men may experience a decrease in testosterone levels.

Mental Health and Its Role in Reproductive Health

1. **The Impact of Stress on Fertility**: Mental health, particularly stress and anxiety, plays a significant role in reproductive health. Chronic stress has been shown to negatively affect hormone levels, leading to irregular menstrual cycles, poor sperm quality, and decreased libido. High levels of stress can also hinder the effectiveness of fertility treatments, such as IVF, by affecting the body's response to hormonal medications.

    - **In Women**: Stress is known to affect the hypothalamic-pituitary-ovarian axis (HPO axis), which regulates hormone production. High cortisol levels, a common result of stress, can suppress reproductive hormones, leading to delayed or absent ovulation. Stress may also contribute to conditions such as endometriosis or polycystic ovary syndrome (PCOS), which are linked to infertility.

- **In Men**: Chronic stress can lead to lower testosterone levels, decreased sperm production, and impaired erectile function. Furthermore, stress may negatively impact sexual performance, making it more difficult for couples to conceive.

2. **Mental Health Disorders and Reproductive Health**: Mental health conditions, such as depression, anxiety, and eating disorders, can also affect reproductive health. For women, depression and anxiety may lead to irregular periods or difficulty conceiving, while eating disorders can disrupt hormone production, leading to infertility. Men with depression may experience a reduced sex drive, erectile dysfunction, and impaired sperm quality.

    - **Addressing Mental Health**: Managing stress and mental health disorders is essential for optimizing reproductive health. Practices such as mindfulness, meditation, yoga, and relaxation techniques can help reduce stress and improve overall well-being. Cognitive behavioral therapy (CBT) and counseling can also be helpful for individuals coping with fertility-related anxiety or depression.
    - **The Role of Support Networks**: Having a strong support network is crucial during times of reproductive health challenges. Emotional support from partners, friends, family, and professional counselors

can help individuals cope with the psychological aspects of fertility struggles, miscarriage, or infertility treatments.

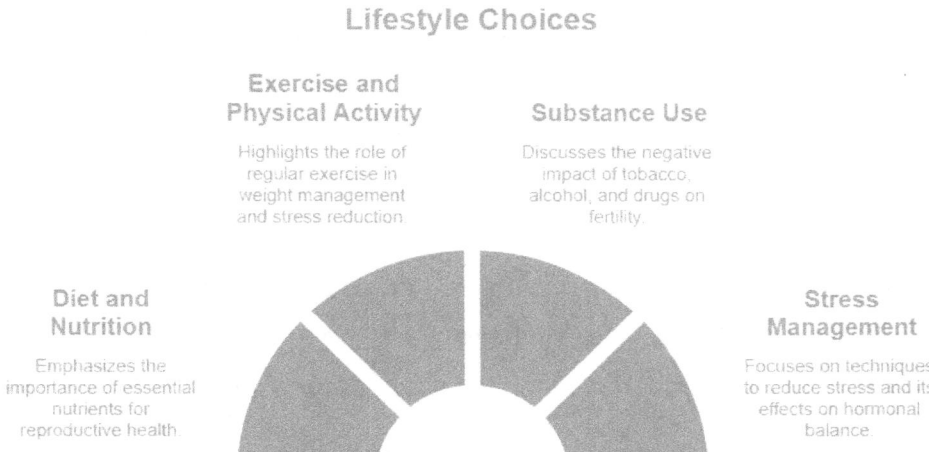

Conclusion

Lifestyle choices have a profound impact on reproductive health, and making positive changes can significantly improve fertility, sexual health, and overall well-being. Smoking, excessive alcohol consumption, and drug use can all detract from reproductive function, while maintaining a healthy weight, staying physically active, and managing mental health can enhance fertility outcomes. The integration of healthy lifestyle choices into daily routines not only supports reproductive health but also contributes to a higher quality of life. By recognizing the powerful connection between lifestyle and reproductive function, individuals can make informed decisions that promote long-term health and fertility.

Chapter 20

Surgical Interventions: When Necessary

Surgical interventions can play a crucial role in the management of reproductive and sexual health conditions. While many conditions can be managed through medical therapies, lifestyle adjustments, and other non-invasive treatments, surgery may become necessary when other options fail or when the condition is severe enough to require a more direct approach. Whether it's for conditions like ovarian cysts, uterine fibroids, prostate issues, or other reproductive disorders, surgery often provides a solution when symptoms become debilitating or when there are significant risks to long-term health and fertility.

This chapter will explore the different types of surgeries used to treat common reproductive and sexual health conditions, the benefits and risks associated with these procedures, and the post-surgical care required for optimal recovery. Additionally, we'll discuss the advancements in surgical techniques, comparing minimally invasive surgeries with traditional methods, to provide a comprehensive understanding of what patients can expect when surgery becomes necessary.

Surgical Procedures for Common Reproductive and Sexual Health Conditions

1. **Ovarian Cysts**: Ovarian cysts are fluid-filled sacs that form on the ovaries, and while many cysts resolve on their own, some may require surgical intervention, particularly if they cause significant pain, grow large, or lead to complications like ovarian torsion (twisting of the ovary) or rupture.

- **Cystectomy**: In cases where the cyst is large or persistent, a cystectomy may be performed. This procedure involves the removal of the cyst without removing the ovary itself. It is commonly done through laparoscopic (minimally invasive) surgery, where small incisions are made in the abdomen, and a camera is inserted to guide the surgeon. Cystectomy preserves ovarian function, allowing for future fertility.

- **Oophorectomy**: In rare cases, when cysts are recurrent or cancerous, the ovary may need to be removed entirely in a procedure called an oophorectomy. This is often done if the cyst poses a significant threat to health, such as with the presence of cancer or advanced endometriosis.

2. **Uterine Fibroids**: Uterine fibroids are benign growths that develop in the muscle wall of the uterus and are a common cause of symptoms like heavy menstrual bleeding, pelvic pain, and reproductive complications. Treatment options for fibroids can range from medication to surgery, with surgery being considered when fibroids are large or cause significant symptoms.

    - **Myomectomy**: A myomectomy is the surgical removal of fibroids from the uterus. This can be done through various methods, including laparotomy (open surgery), laparoscopy (minimally invasive surgery), or hysteroscopy (a procedure in which instruments are inserted through the cervix). Myomectomy is often preferred for women who want to preserve their fertility, as it allows them to retain their uterus while removing the fibroids.

- **Hysterectomy**: In cases where the fibroids are numerous or cause severe symptoms that do not respond to other treatments, a hysterectomy (removal of the uterus) may be recommended. This procedure is typically a last resort for women who do not wish to preserve their fertility or when other treatment options have been exhausted.

3. **Prostate Issues**: Prostate problems, including benign prostatic hyperplasia (BPH), prostate cancer, and prostatitis, can all lead to urinary symptoms, pain, and sexual dysfunction. Surgery may be indicated when non-invasive treatments, such as medications, do not provide relief or when the condition is particularly severe.

    - **Transurethral Resection of the Prostate (TURP)**: TURP is the most common surgical procedure for BPH, a condition in which the prostate enlarges and obstructs the flow of urine. During the procedure, the surgeon removes part of the prostate using a special instrument inserted through the urethra, which avoids the need for external incisions. TURP provides relief from urinary symptoms and improves quality of life for many men.

    - **Prostatectomy**: In cases of prostate cancer or advanced BPH, a prostatectomy, the removal of the prostate gland, may be recommended. This can be done through open surgery or laparoscopic (robot-assisted) surgery. A radical prostatectomy may be necessary when the cancer is localized and has not spread to surrounding tissues, whereas a simpler prostatectomy may be considered for benign conditions.

- **Laser Surgery**: For men with BPH, laser surgery is another minimally invasive option. Laser therapy uses high-energy light to vaporize or shrink the prostate tissue, which can improve urine flow and relieve symptoms without the need for traditional surgery.

Minimally Invasive vs. Traditional Surgery

Advancements in surgical techniques have made it possible to treat many reproductive and sexual health conditions through minimally invasive procedures. These procedures generally offer quicker recovery times, reduced risk of complications, and less scarring compared to traditional open surgery. However, there are situations where traditional surgery may still be necessary.

1. **Minimally Invasive Surgery**: Minimally invasive surgery involves using small incisions, often just a few millimeters in size, through which the surgeon can insert a camera and special surgical instruments to perform the procedure. Some common types of minimally invasive surgery include laparoscopy and robotic-assisted surgery. These procedures have revolutionized the way reproductive and sexual health conditions are treated.

    - **Benefits**:
        - Shorter hospital stays and faster recovery times.
        - Less postoperative pain and scarring.
        - Reduced risk of infection and complications.
        - A faster return to daily activities and work.
    - **Conditions Treated**:
        - Ovarian cyst removal.

- Myomectomy (removal of fibroids).
- Hysterectomy (in certain cases).
- Prostate surgeries (e.g., TURP, prostatectomy).
  - **Technological Advances**: Robotic-assisted surgery, a form of minimally invasive surgery, provides the surgeon with enhanced precision and control. With robotic systems like the da Vinci Surgical System, surgeons can perform complex procedures with a higher degree of accuracy, often leading to better outcomes for patients.

2. **Traditional (Open) Surgery**: Traditional surgery, involving larger incisions and more direct access to the affected organ, is still used in certain situations, especially when minimally invasive surgery is not feasible or when the condition requires more extensive intervention.
   - **Benefits**:
     - Better access for complex surgeries.
     - Suitable for larger fibroids or advanced prostate cancer.
     - In cases where a surgeon needs to remove a large amount of tissue or when other methods have failed.
   - **Conditions Treated**:
     - Large uterine fibroids.
     - Advanced prostate cancer.
     - Severe cases of endometriosis or ovarian cysts.
   - **Risks**:

- Longer recovery times.
- Higher risk of infection.
- Increased blood loss and scarring.

Recovery and Post-Surgical Care

The recovery process after surgery varies depending on the type of procedure performed, the patient's overall health, and the surgical approach. However, all surgeries require careful monitoring and post-operative care to ensure optimal healing and minimize the risk of complications.

1. **Minimally Invasive Surgery Recovery**:
    - **Hospital Stay**: Most minimally invasive surgeries require a shorter hospital stay, often just a day or two, depending on the patient's condition and the complexity of the procedure.
    - **Recovery Time**: The recovery time is typically quicker than traditional surgery, with many patients able to return to normal activities within a few weeks. Light exercise may be allowed after 2-4 weeks, but full physical activity or heavy lifting may need to be avoided for longer.
    - **Post-Operative Care**: Patients are often advised to take pain medication as needed, follow up with their surgeon for regular check-ups, and adhere to any specific guidelines for wound care or activity restrictions. Some patients may be given instructions on pelvic floor exercises, particularly after procedures like a myomectomy or hysterectomy.

2. **Traditional Surgery Recovery**:

- **Hospital Stay**: For traditional surgeries, such as an open hysterectomy or prostatectomy, the hospital stay is generally longer, typically 3-5 days, depending on the patient's health and the complexity of the procedure.

- **Recovery Time**: Recovery can take longer, with most patients requiring 6-8 weeks to return to normal activities. It's essential to follow all post-surgical instructions, including avoiding strenuous activity and managing pain effectively.

- **Post-Operative Care**: Patients may experience more significant pain and require more extensive wound care. Depending on the surgery, the surgeon may recommend a rehabilitation plan, including physical therapy, to restore normal function and strength. Patients must also be monitored for complications such as infection, blood clots, or bleeding.

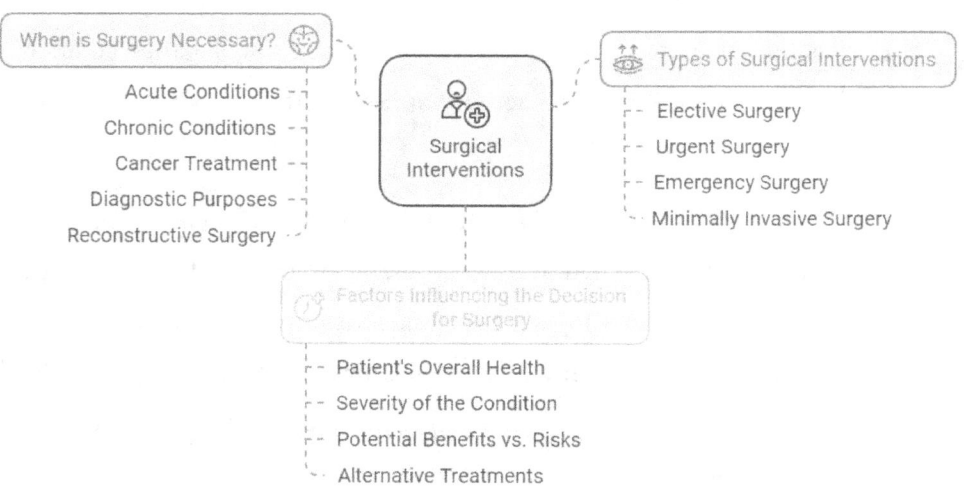

Conclusion

Surgical intervention plays a vital role in the treatment of many reproductive and sexual health conditions, offering relief from symptoms, preserving fertility, and improving quality of life. Whether it is the removal of ovarian cysts, treatment of uterine fibroids, or addressing prostate issues, surgery can provide a path toward better health when other treatments are not effective. Understanding the different surgical options, including minimally invasive versus traditional approaches, and knowing what to expect during recovery, can help patients make informed decisions about their health. By working closely with healthcare providers, individuals can choose the best surgical approach for their specific needs and take the necessary steps to ensure a smooth and successful recovery.

Chapter 21

Fertility Treatments and Assisted Reproductive Technologies (ART)

Introduction: The Evolution of Reproductive Medicine

Advances in reproductive medicine have revolutionized the way healthcare providers address infertility and reproductive challenges. For many individuals and couples, these breakthroughs have offered hope when faced with the emotional and physical burden of infertility. Assisted Reproductive Technologies (ART) encompass a range of medical interventions and treatments designed to assist with conception. From in vitro fertilization (IVF) to fertility preservation techniques, ART has significantly enhanced the success rates of conception for individuals who experience difficulty in becoming pregnant naturally. Furthermore, emerging technologies such as egg and sperm donation, as well as surrogacy, have expanded family-building options for individuals who cannot carry a pregnancy themselves or who face other fertility challenges.

In this chapter, we will explore the various types of ART, the scientific principles behind these methods, their success rates, and the ethical and social considerations that come with these advancements. Whether it's IVF, cryopreservation, or surrogacy, understanding the options available allows individuals and couples to make informed decisions about their reproductive futures.

In Vitro Fertilization (IVF): The Pinnacle of Assisted Reproductive Technology

In vitro fertilization (IVF) is one of the most well-known and widely used ART methods. IVF involves the fertilization of an egg outside of the body in a laboratory dish, followed by the implantation of the fertilized embryo into the uterus. This process offers a solution for individuals or couples facing various infertility challenges, such as blocked fallopian tubes, male infertility, endometriosis, or unexplained infertility.

1. **The IVF Process:** The IVF procedure begins with ovarian stimulation. Fertility medications are administered to stimulate the ovaries to produce multiple eggs, as opposed to the single egg typically released during a natural menstrual cycle. Once the eggs are mature, they are retrieved through a minimally invasive procedure known as egg retrieval. A needle is inserted through the vaginal wall, and under ultrasound guidance, the eggs are collected.

After egg retrieval, the eggs are fertilized in the laboratory using sperm, either from the male partner or a donor. The fertilized eggs are cultured for a few days, typically 3 to 5 days, to allow them to develop into embryos. The embryos are then assessed for quality, and the best quality embryos are selected for transfer into the woman's uterus. Any surplus embryos may be frozen for future use.

2. **Success Rates:** Success rates for IVF vary based on a variety of factors, including the woman's age, the cause of infertility, the quality of the eggs and sperm, and the expertise of the fertility clinic. On average, the success rate of IVF tends to decrease with maternal age, with women under 35 having the highest success rates, typically between 40-50% per cycle. For women over 40, success rates drop significantly, often below 20%. It is important to note that IVF success also depends on how many embryos are transferred and whether preimplantation genetic testing is used to identify genetic abnormalities in embryos.

While IVF is not always successful on the first attempt, multiple cycles may increase the chances of pregnancy. Clinics may use strategies such as embryo freezing, egg donation, or the use of gestational carriers to improve outcomes for individuals who do not have success with a single IVF cycle.

Cryopreservation and Fertility Preservation

Fertility preservation is a crucial aspect of reproductive medicine, offering individuals the opportunity to preserve their fertility for future use. Cryopreservation—the freezing of eggs, sperm, and embryos—is a vital technique that allows individuals to store reproductive material to delay parenthood or safeguard fertility in cases where medical treatments might affect reproductive function.

1. **Egg Freezing:** Egg freezing has become an increasingly popular option for women who wish to delay childbearing due to personal or medical reasons. The process involves stimulating the ovaries to produce multiple eggs, as in IVF, followed by egg retrieval and freezing for later use. This technique is particularly valuable for women diagnosed with conditions such as cancer, which require treatments like chemotherapy that may affect fertility. Egg freezing also offers a viable option for women who wish to preserve their fertility while pursuing career goals or waiting for the right time to start a family.

    - **Success Rates and Considerations**: The success of egg freezing depends on the age of the woman at the time of egg retrieval. Younger women (typically under 35) have higher success rates with frozen eggs, as egg quality diminishes with age. For women considering this option, it is essential to understand the potential for multiple cycles of egg retrieval to maximize the number of eggs available for future use.

2. **Sperm Freezing:** Sperm freezing is a similar process in which sperm is collected and preserved for future use. This technique is commonly used by men undergoing medical treatments such as chemotherapy, which may impact sperm production. It also offers an option for men who wish to delay fatherhood or have fertility preservation concerns due to aging or lifestyle factors.

    o **Success Rates**: Sperm freezing has a high success rate, as sperm can be stored indefinitely with little degradation in quality. Success rates for pregnancy depend on factors such as sperm quality at the time of freezing, the woman's age, and the method of insemination used during future ART cycles.

3. **Embryo Freezing:** Embryo freezing is an option for couples undergoing IVF who have surplus embryos after a successful fertilization cycle. These embryos can be cryopreserved and used in subsequent IVF cycles if needed. Embryo freezing offers a higher success rate than egg or sperm freezing because embryos are already fertilized and can be directly transferred to the uterus.

    o **Considerations**: Embryo freezing requires a decision to be made regarding the use of eggs and sperm from the same cycle. For individuals undergoing IVF who have embryos available for freezing, it provides the opportunity to attempt pregnancy in the future without having to undergo the full IVF process again.

Surrogacy: An Alternative Path to Parenthood

Surrogacy is another important option in the realm of reproductive medicine, allowing individuals and couples to have a child when they cannot carry a pregnancy themselves. Surrogacy involves a woman (the surrogate) who carries a pregnancy for another person or couple, usually due to medical reasons such as uterine abnormalities, severe infertility, or other health issues that prevent pregnancy.

1. **Types of Surrogacy:**

    - **Traditional Surrogacy**: In traditional surrogacy, the surrogate mother is also the biological mother of the child. The surrogate's egg is fertilized by the intended father's sperm or donor sperm through artificial insemination. This type of surrogacy is less common today due to the legal complexities and emotional challenges it presents.

    - **Gestational Surrogacy**: Gestational surrogacy involves the use of the intended mother's or a donor's eggs, which are fertilized via IVF, and the resulting embryo is implanted into the surrogate's uterus. The surrogate has no genetic relationship to the child. Gestational surrogacy is the preferred method and offers greater legal clarity, as the child is genetically linked to the intended parents.

2. **Legal and Ethical Considerations**: Surrogacy presents various ethical and legal challenges that vary by region and country. In some places, surrogacy is tightly regulated, while in others, it may be prohibited or poorly defined. Intended parents must navigate the complex legal landscape to ensure that the surrogate's rights, as well as the intended parents' rights, are protected. Legal contracts are typically used to outline responsibilities, compensation, and the parental rights of the intended parents.

- **Compensation and Relationship Dynamics**: Surrogates may be compensated for their time, effort, and medical expenses, and this financial arrangement can vary based on the country and whether the surrogacy is commercial or altruistic. The emotional and psychological impact of surrogacy can also be profound, requiring clear communication, counseling, and support for all parties involved.

3. **Success Rates of Surrogacy**: The success of gestational surrogacy largely depends on the age of the intended mother or the egg donor, as well as the quality of the embryos created during IVF. Surrogacy has a relatively high success rate compared to other ART methods, but the process can still take several months or years, especially if multiple IVF attempts are needed or if a suitable surrogate is not available immediately.

Egg and Sperm Donation: Expanding Reproductive Options

Egg and sperm donation is an ART option that allows individuals and couples to build their families when they are unable to conceive with their own reproductive material. This option is commonly used in cases where one partner has fertility issues, such as low egg quality or male infertility, or when both partners are infertile.

1. **Egg Donation**: Egg donation involves the use of eggs from a donor, typically a young woman under the age of 30, to assist women who cannot produce viable eggs of their own. Egg donors are carefully screened for health, genetic conditions, and lifestyle factors. The donated eggs are fertilized with the intended father's sperm or donor sperm via IVF, and the resulting embryos are implanted into the intended mother's uterus.

- **Success Rates**: Egg donation has a high success rate, particularly for women over 40, as the quality of the eggs is more likely to be optimal in younger donors. Women who use egg donation typically have success rates similar to women who are in their 20s or early 30s.

2. **Sperm Donation**: Sperm donation allows individuals or couples who face male infertility, sperm quality issues, or those who are single or in same-sex relationships to use donor sperm for conception. The sperm is collected, processed, and stored in sperm banks, from where it can be selected by the intended parent(s). The sperm is then used in ART procedures such as intrauterine insemination (IUI) or IVF.

    - **Success Rates**: Success rates for sperm donation depend on the type of ART used, the age of the woman receiving the sperm, and the quality of the sperm. Sperm donation offers a high success rate in cases of male infertility.

Exploring the Spectrum of Fertility Treatments

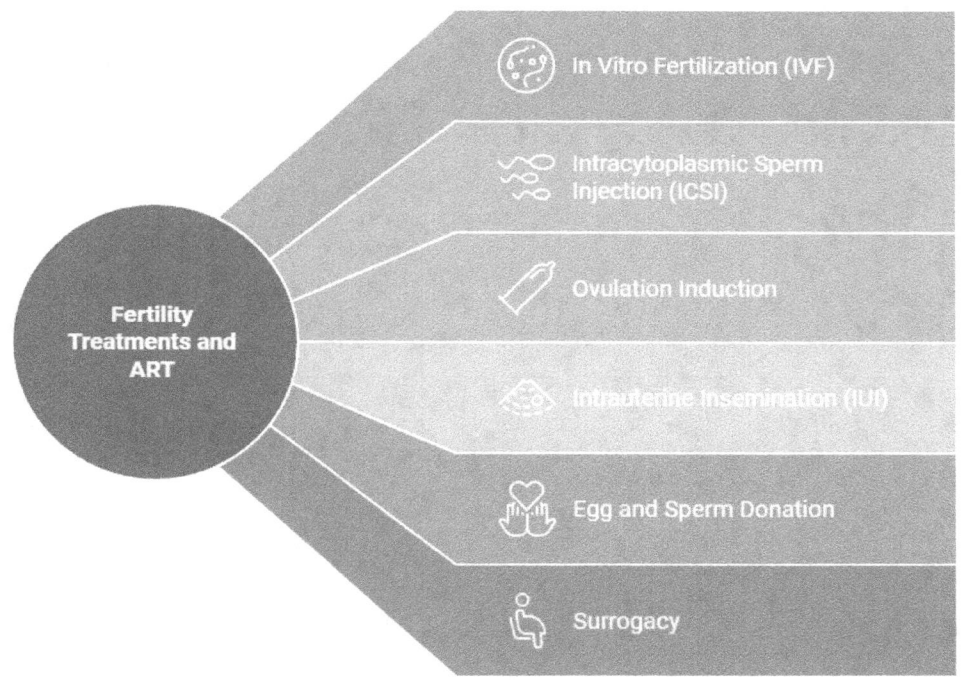

Conclusion

Advances in fertility treatments and assisted reproductive technologies have transformed the way individuals and couples approach reproductive challenges. IVF, cryopreservation, surrogacy, egg and sperm donation, and other ART options have given rise to new possibilities for family-building, ensuring that people can create families even in the face of medical barriers. With ongoing advancements in technology and research, the future of reproductive medicine holds even greater promise, offering individuals more personalized and accessible options for achieving parenthood. As these treatments continue to evolve, it is essential to stay informed and empowered by understanding the various options, success rates, and ethical considerations associated with ART.

Chapter 22

The Future of Male and Female Infertility Treatments

Introduction: Shaping the Future of Reproductive Medicine

Infertility has long been a challenging and emotionally complex issue for individuals and couples who dream of becoming parents. However, with the advancement of medical science and technology, fertility treatments have dramatically evolved, offering new hope and opportunities for those struggling with reproductive health. From in vitro fertilization (IVF) to egg freezing, assisted reproductive technologies (ART) have made significant strides in improving success rates and helping people overcome infertility. But as the field of reproductive medicine continues to grow, emerging technologies and cutting-edge research are bringing even more innovative solutions to the table.

In this chapter, we will explore the future of male and female infertility treatments, focusing on the latest advancements that are set to revolutionize the way infertility is diagnosed and treated. This includes groundbreaking technologies such as gene therapy, stem cell research, and personalized fertility treatments. These innovations offer the promise of not only improving treatment outcomes but also changing the very landscape of how infertility is understood and managed.

Emerging Technologies in Fertility Treatment

The future of fertility treatment lies in the continuous development of new technologies that enhance the accuracy, effectiveness, and accessibility of care. From advanced genetic screening techniques to improvements in IVF methods, emerging technologies are paving the way for more efficient and successful treatments.

1. **Artificial Intelligence (AI) in Fertility Diagnosis and Treatment**: One of the most exciting areas in reproductive medicine is the use of artificial intelligence (AI) to improve fertility outcomes. AI can be used to analyze vast amounts of data, including patient history, test results, and even embryo development, to make more accurate predictions about the chances of successful conception. AI-driven algorithms are being incorporated into fertility clinics to enhance decision-making regarding the best course of treatment, such as the selection of the most viable embryos during IVF or the optimal time for egg retrieval.

AI's role in fertility is also extending to personalized care, where treatments are tailored to the individual needs of patients. AI can identify patterns in a patient's fertility history and adjust treatment plans to maximize success rates. Additionally, AI-powered platforms can track ovulation cycles and fertility windows more precisely, enabling couples to time intercourse or ART procedures for optimal chances of conception.

2. **Gene Editing and Gene Therapy**: Gene therapy is an emerging frontier that could revolutionize fertility treatments, particularly for individuals facing genetic disorders that impact fertility. One of the most significant breakthroughs in this area is the development of CRISPR (Clustered Regularly Interspaced Short Palindromic Repeats), a technology that allows scientists to edit genes with high precision. With CRISPR, researchers are exploring the possibility of correcting genetic mutations that cause infertility or genetic disorders in embryos before implantation.

   - **Gene Editing for Inherited Conditions**: For individuals who carry genetic mutations that could lead to inherited diseases (such as cystic fibrosis or sickle cell anemia), gene editing could offer a way to prevent the transmission of these conditions to offspring. By editing the genes of embryos at the earliest stages, researchers hope to eliminate the risk of passing on genetic disorders, significantly reducing the likelihood of miscarriage and genetic complications.

- **Improving Sperm and Egg Quality**: Gene therapy also holds promise in improving the quality of eggs and sperm in individuals experiencing age-related infertility. By targeting and repairing the genetic material within sperm and eggs, researchers could increase fertility potential, helping those who may otherwise have difficulty conceiving due to poor egg quality or sperm motility.

3. **3D Printing of Ovarian and Testicular Tissue**: In an era where bioengineering and biotechnology are advancing rapidly, scientists are exploring the possibility of 3D printing functional reproductive tissues. For women who undergo treatments like chemotherapy and experience ovarian failure, 3D-printed ovarian tissues could offer a potential solution. These tissues could be used to restore hormone production, fertility, or even the ability to carry a pregnancy in the future.

Similarly, 3D printing techniques may be used to create testicular tissues for men who have low sperm production or other fertility issues. This could lead to the development of personalized, biologically compatible tissues that support fertility. Though still in the experimental stages, these technologies have the potential to transform the landscape of infertility treatments in the coming decades.

Stem Cell Research and Its Role in Fertility

Stem cell research has long been a topic of intense interest, especially in the realm of reproductive medicine. Stem cells have the unique ability to develop into any type of cell in the body, making them an invaluable resource for regenerative medicine. In fertility treatments, stem cells are being investigated for their potential to restore fertility, repair damaged reproductive organs, and regenerate eggs or sperm.

1. **Stem Cells for Egg and Sperm Production**: One of the most groundbreaking areas of stem cell research is the ability to create eggs and sperm from other cell types. Researchers have already successfully generated egg-like cells and sperm-like cells from stem cells in laboratory settings. The ability to generate viable eggs and sperm from a person's own stem cells could offer a solution for individuals with infertility due to age, genetic factors, or medical treatments that damage the reproductive system.

    - **For Women**: Female fertility declines with age, primarily because of the limited number of eggs available in the ovaries. Stem cell-based therapies could regenerate ovarian tissues and produce fresh eggs, enabling women to conceive later in life without relying on egg donation or IVF. Researchers are also working on creating ovarian tissue that could be transplanted back into women's bodies, providing a way to restore fertility following treatments like chemotherapy or ovarian surgery.

    - **For Men**: Male infertility, often caused by low sperm count or poor sperm quality, could be addressed through stem cell technology as well. By creating sperm from stem cells, scientists may be able to offer new hope to men who are unable to produce viable sperm. This breakthrough could also be useful in cases where a man's sperm quality is compromised by medical conditions, aging, or lifestyle factors.

2. **Regeneration of Reproductive Organs**: Stem cell therapy may also be used to regenerate damaged reproductive organs, such as the ovaries or testes. For women with conditions like premature ovarian failure or polycystic ovary syndrome (PCOS), stem cells could offer a potential solution for restoring ovarian function. In men, stem cell therapies may aid in regenerating the testes, thereby restoring sperm production and hormone levels. While this field is still in its early stages, the potential for stem cells to address a variety of fertility issues is enormous.

Personalized Fertility Solutions: Tailoring Treatments to the Individual

One of the most promising trends in the future of infertility treatments is the move toward personalized care. Personalized medicine involves customizing treatment plans based on an individual's unique genetic makeup, medical history, and lifestyle factors. In the context of fertility, personalized solutions aim to improve outcomes by providing treatments that are specifically tailored to the needs of the patient.

1. **Genetic Testing for Personalized Fertility Plans**: Genetic testing is becoming increasingly common in fertility clinics. By analyzing an individual's DNA, healthcare providers can gain valuable insights into their reproductive health, including their risk for certain fertility-related conditions. For example, testing for genetic mutations that could impact egg or sperm quality or predispose individuals to conditions like endometriosis can guide clinicians in developing a more targeted and effective treatment plan.

    o **Genomic Sequencing of Embryos**: Preimplantation genetic testing (PGT) is already a routine part of IVF for many patients, but future advances in genomic sequencing could allow for even more detailed analysis of embryos before implantation. This may allow for the identification of genetic diseases, chromosomal abnormalities, and even complex traits that affect the likelihood of successful pregnancy. Personalized IVF cycles based on genetic data could optimize outcomes for patients.

2. **Tailored IVF Protocols**: IVF protocols, such as the medications and hormonal treatments used to stimulate the ovaries, can be customized based on a woman's individual response to treatment. Personalized IVF may involve tailoring the treatment based on factors such as ovarian reserve, age, lifestyle, and the underlying cause of infertility. This ensures that each patient receives the most effective and appropriate treatment, increasing the chances of success while minimizing the risk of complications.

3. **Lifestyle Integration**: Another key aspect of personalized fertility treatments involves addressing lifestyle factors that can affect reproductive health. Future treatments will likely integrate nutrition, exercise, mental health support, and other factors into personalized fertility plans. For example, individualized diet plans that address hormonal imbalances, stress reduction techniques, and physical therapy may be included as part of fertility treatment. By addressing the whole person rather than just the reproductive organs, personalized fertility solutions have the potential to significantly improve outcomes.

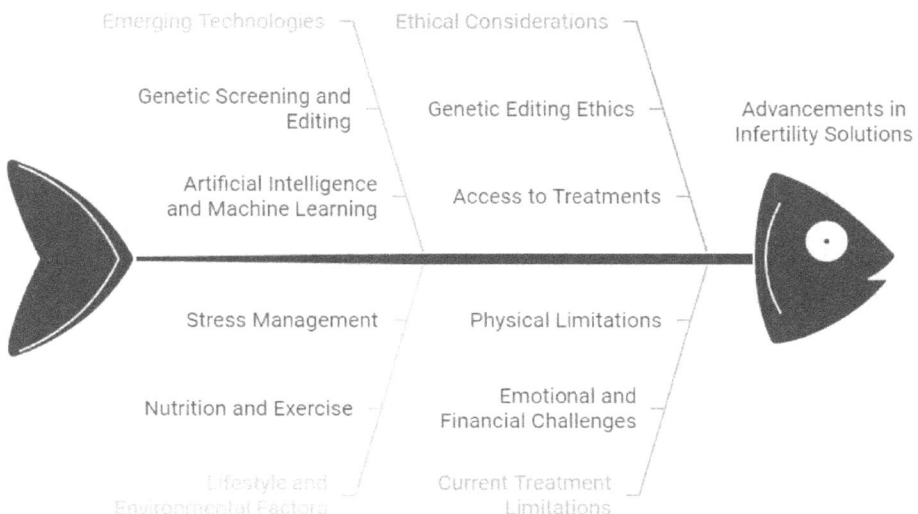

Conclusion

The future of male and female infertility treatments is incredibly promising, with emerging technologies and research offering new possibilities for individuals and couples struggling with fertility. From AI-powered fertility diagnosis to gene therapy and stem cell treatments, the landscape of reproductive medicine is evolving rapidly. These advancements provide new hope for people facing infertility due to age, medical conditions, or other factors that once seemed insurmountable.

While these innovations are still being explored and developed, the potential for groundbreaking breakthroughs in reproductive health is limitless. As technology continues to progress and research uncovers new insights into the complex biology of fertility, the future of fertility treatments will likely be more personalized, more effective, and more accessible, helping people achieve their dreams of parenthood in ways that were once unimaginable.

Chapter 23

Genomic and Personalized Medicine in Reproductive Health

The rapid advances in genomic medicine and personalized healthcare have significantly transformed the field of reproductive medicine. At the heart of these advancements is genetic testing, which has the potential to dramatically influence fertility treatments, pregnancy outcomes, and even the way we approach conditions that affect reproductive health. The ability to examine an individual's genetic makeup and tailor medical care to their specific needs is a groundbreaking development that could change the way we diagnose, prevent, and treat infertility and related disorders.

Genomic and personalized medicine promises to make reproductive care more precise, individualized, and effective. However, with these advancements come important ethical questions and challenges that need to be addressed. In this chapter, we will explore how genetic testing is being used to improve reproductive health, how it impacts fertility and pregnancy outcomes, and the ethical considerations surrounding these powerful technologies.

The Role of Genetic Testing in Fertility and Reproductive Health

Genetic testing plays an increasingly important role in diagnosing and managing infertility. As scientists learn more about the human genome and the intricate biological processes that regulate fertility, they are uncovering genetic factors that influence reproductive health. Genetic testing can identify mutations, variations, and inherited conditions that may prevent conception or lead to pregnancy complications. By understanding these genetic factors, healthcare providers can tailor treatments to optimize fertility, reduce the risk of genetic disorders, and enhance the likelihood of a healthy pregnancy.

1. **Genetic Screening for Inherited Disorders**: One of the most important uses of genetic testing in reproductive health is the identification of inherited genetic disorders that can affect offspring. For couples who are carriers of specific genetic conditions, such as cystic fibrosis, sickle cell anemia, or Tay-Sachs disease, genetic screening can help determine the risk of passing these conditions to their children. Carrier screening, which can be done before conception or during pregnancy, identifies whether both parents carry the same genetic mutation, which increases the likelihood that their child may inherit the disorder.

By performing pre-conception genetic screening, couples can gain valuable insight into their risk of having a child with a genetic disorder. If both partners are found to be carriers of the same genetic condition, options such as preimplantation genetic testing (PGT) during IVF can be used to select embryos without the inherited condition, thus reducing the likelihood of passing on genetic diseases. This type of genetic testing allows for informed decision-making and provides an opportunity to minimize the risk of genetic conditions.

2. **Chromosomal Abnormalities and IVF**: Chromosomal abnormalities, such as Down syndrome or other conditions caused by an extra or missing chromosome, are a common cause of miscarriage, infertility, or birth defects. Advances in genetic testing, particularly in the form of preimplantation genetic testing for aneuploidy (PGT-A), are allowing doctors to screen embryos created through in vitro fertilization (IVF) for chromosomal abnormalities before they are implanted in the uterus.

PGT-A analyzes the chromosomes of embryos to detect any structural or numerical abnormalities that might lead to unsuccessful implantation, early pregnancy loss, or developmental issues. By identifying the healthiest embryos, doctors can increase the chances of a successful pregnancy and reduce the risk of genetic disorders. This form of genetic testing offers couples greater control over their reproductive journey, helping them avoid the heartache of miscarriage and the uncertainty of unknown genetic conditions.

3. **Genetic Testing for Male Infertility**: Male infertility, often caused by low sperm count, poor sperm motility, or abnormal sperm morphology, can also be influenced by genetic factors. Recent studies have revealed that certain genetic mutations or chromosomal issues can contribute to male infertility. Genetic tests for male infertility focus on evaluating the Y chromosome, which carries genes responsible for sperm production. One of the most notable tests is the assessment of Y chromosome microdeletions, which are associated with reduced sperm production and infertility.

Identifying these genetic markers in men with unexplained infertility can offer valuable insights into treatment options. In some cases, men with genetic causes of infertility may be eligible for sperm retrieval techniques such as testicular sperm extraction (TESE) or other assisted reproductive technologies (ART). In cases where sperm is not available or viable, sperm donation may be considered. By understanding the genetic causes of male infertility, healthcare providers can develop more personalized treatment plans that improve the chances of successful fertilization and conception.

4. **Fertility Preservation and Genetic Counseling**: Fertility preservation is another area where genetic testing is playing a crucial role. For individuals undergoing treatments that could affect fertility, such as chemotherapy,

radiation, or gender-affirming treatments, genetic testing can help identify any risks associated with fertility preservation. For example, certain genetic conditions may affect the quality or quantity of eggs or sperm, potentially limiting the success of fertility preservation procedures like egg or sperm banking.

Genetic counseling can also assist individuals considering fertility preservation by providing them with a comprehensive understanding of their fertility potential and any associated risks. By examining family history and genetic predispositions, counselors can help individuals make informed decisions about preserving their fertility and choosing the most appropriate methods for doing so.

Personalized Medicine: Tailoring Fertility Treatments

As the field of genetics advances, fertility treatments are becoming more personalized, focusing not just on the condition being treated but also on the individual's genetic makeup. Personalized medicine takes into account a person's unique genetic profile, environmental factors, lifestyle, and medical history to develop a treatment plan that is specifically suited to their needs.

1. **Genetic-Based IVF Protocols**: One of the key areas where personalized medicine is making a difference is in IVF treatment protocols. Traditionally, IVF involves a standard regimen of hormonal stimulation to induce egg production, followed by egg retrieval, fertilization, and embryo transfer. However, not all patients respond to IVF in the same way. Some women may require higher or lower doses of medication, or may benefit from different types of stimulation protocols based on their genetic profile.

Recent advancements in personalized medicine are allowing fertility specialists to tailor IVF protocols based on genetic tests. For example, genetic screening can help determine a woman's response to ovarian stimulation by identifying specific genetic variations that affect hormone metabolism and egg quality. This ensures that the treatment plan is optimized for the individual's needs, increasing the chances of a successful pregnancy while minimizing side effects and complications.

2. **Pharmacogenetics in Fertility Treatments**: Pharmacogenetics is the study of how genes influence an individual's response to medications. In fertility treatments, pharmacogenetic testing can be used to determine how a patient's body will metabolize certain fertility drugs, such as gonadotropins or progesterone. By understanding the genetic factors that influence drug absorption and effectiveness, doctors can prescribe more targeted medications that will have the desired effect, improving the overall success of fertility treatments.

3. **Personalized Sperm and Egg Selection**: The future of reproductive medicine may involve more personalized approaches to sperm and egg selection. In the case of sperm donation, genetic testing can identify sperm that carry fewer genetic mutations, which may improve the quality of the embryo and increase the chances of successful fertilization. Similarly, the selection of eggs for IVF could be optimized based on genetic screening, identifying those with the highest quality and the least likelihood of chromosomal abnormalities.

Ethical Considerations of Genetic Interventions

While the potential of genetic testing and personalized medicine to improve reproductive health is immense, it also raises important ethical considerations. These include questions about privacy, the potential for genetic discrimination, and the ethical implications of selecting for certain traits or eliminating genetic conditions.

1. **Genetic Privacy and Consent**: Genetic testing involves sensitive personal data that could have far-reaching implications for individuals and their families. As such, ensuring the privacy of genetic information is of paramount importance. Genetic tests for fertility or pregnancy-related conditions must be conducted with the informed consent of the individual, and patients should be fully aware of how their genetic data will be used and stored.

Ethical concerns also arise regarding who has access to genetic data. For example, employers or insurance companies might use genetic information to make decisions about hiring or coverage, leading to potential discrimination. This makes it crucial to have strong regulations in place to protect against genetic discrimination and ensure that individuals' rights are safeguarded.

2. **Designer Babies and Genetic Selection**: Another controversial issue surrounding genetic testing and interventions is the possibility of "designer babies." While current genetic screening primarily focuses on preventing genetic disorders, future advancements could make it possible to select embryos based on desirable traits, such as intelligence, physical appearance, or athletic ability. This raises ethical concerns about the potential for eugenics and the creation of a societal divide between those who can afford genetic modifications and those who cannot.

The idea of selecting for non-medical traits challenges our notions of human diversity and autonomy. Many ethicists argue that while we should aim to prevent serious genetic diseases, the idea of choosing traits like eye color or intelligence should be approached with caution, as it could lead to unintended social and ethical consequences.

3. **Reproductive Equity and Accessibility**: While genetic testing and personalized medicine hold great promise, they are not universally accessible. The high cost of genetic testing, IVF, and other assisted reproductive technologies can create barriers to access for many individuals, particularly those from low-income backgrounds or marginalized communities. Ensuring that advances in reproductive medicine are accessible to all people, regardless of their socioeconomic status, is an important ethical consideration as the field moves forward.

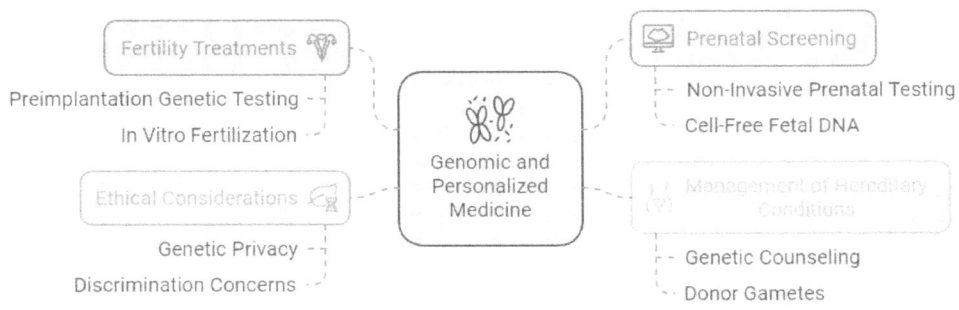

Conclusion

Genomic and personalized medicine has the potential to transform the field of reproductive health, offering individuals and couples new opportunities to understand their fertility, optimize their chances of conception, and avoid genetic disorders. From genetic screening and IVF to pharmacogenetics and personalized treatment plans, the future of fertility care is more individualized and effective than ever before.

However, with these advancements come significant ethical considerations. As we continue to explore the potential of genetic interventions in reproductive health, it is essential that we navigate the complex ethical landscape with care, ensuring that these technologies are used responsibly, fairly, and with respect for individual autonomy and privacy.

As research and technology continue to evolve, genomic medicine will undoubtedly play an increasingly important role in reproductive health, offering new solutions and possibilities for those struggling with infertility or genetic conditions. But with great power comes great responsibility, and it is essential that we strike a balance between innovation and ethical considerations to ensure that these advancements benefit all individuals, without compromising our core values.

Chapter 24

Adolescent Reproductive Health

Introduction: The Foundation of Reproductive Health

Adolescence is a transformative period in human development, marked by profound physical, emotional, and social changes. Among these changes, the maturation of the reproductive system plays a central role, as young individuals transition from childhood to adulthood. The onset of puberty signals the beginning of these developmental processes, influencing not only fertility but also sexual health, emotional well-being, and identity. Understanding adolescent reproductive health is critical to promoting long-term wellness and ensuring that young people are equipped with the knowledge and resources they need to navigate the challenges of sexual and reproductive health.

In this chapter, we will explore the biological and physiological changes that occur during puberty, address the importance of sexual health education, and discuss the preventive strategies that can help adolescents maintain their reproductive health throughout these formative years.

Puberty and the Development of the Reproductive System

Puberty is the time in an individual's life when their body undergoes significant hormonal and physiological changes that enable sexual maturity and reproductive capability. These changes are driven by the activation of the hypothalamic-pituitary-gonadal axis, which triggers the production of sex hormones like estrogen in females and testosterone in males. Puberty typically begins between the ages of 8 and 14 for girls and 9 and 15 for boys, though the exact timing can vary.

Changes in Girls:

1. **Breast Development and Menstruation:** One of the first signs of puberty in girls is the development of breast buds. This occurs as the body begins producing estrogen, leading to the growth of glandular tissue in the breasts. Alongside breast development, girls will experience the growth of pubic and underarm hair. The onset of menstruation, known as menarche, marks the official beginning of reproductive capability. Menstruation typically occurs around two to three years after the onset of puberty, signaling that a girl's body is capable of ovulation and reproduction.

2. **Physical Growth:** Puberty in girls is also marked by a rapid increase in height and changes in body composition. This includes the widening of the hips and an increase in body fat, particularly in the breasts, hips, and thighs. These changes are not only necessary for future pregnancy and childbirth but are also indicators of the body's growing sexual maturity.

3. **Psychological and Emotional Changes:** The hormonal fluctuations associated with puberty can lead to emotional changes as well. Adolescent girls may experience mood swings, heightened sensitivity, and a developing sense of body image. These changes are part of the natural process of becoming an adult and are often influenced by peer pressure, societal expectations, and personal experiences. Navigating these emotional shifts is essential for maintaining mental health during this period.

Changes in Boys:

1. **Testicular Enlargement and Growth of Pubic Hair:** For boys, puberty is marked by the enlargement of the testes and the growth of pubic and facial hair. Testosterone production increases, triggering the growth of the penis and the deepening of the voice. These physical changes occur gradually, and

like girls, boys will experience a surge in height as well as a broadening of the shoulders and chest.

2. **Sperm Production:** During puberty, the testes begin to produce sperm, which is the first sign that a boy is capable of reproduction. The first ejaculation, often experienced in early adolescence, marks the onset of sperm production and sexual maturity. The appearance of nocturnal emissions, or "wet dreams," is a natural part of this process.

3. **Muscle Development and Physical Strength:** As testosterone levels rise, boys will experience an increase in muscle mass and strength. These physical changes are crucial for male sexual maturation and the ability to reproduce.

4. **Psychological and Emotional Development:** Much like their female counterparts, adolescent boys experience emotional and psychological growth during puberty. This includes the development of self-identity, the formation of sexual preferences, and the desire for independence from parents and caregivers. Peer relationships often become central to this stage of life, and boys may face pressures related to masculinity, body image, and sexual performance.

Addressing Sexual Health Education

Comprehensive sexual health education is crucial during adolescence to help young people navigate the complexities of puberty and sexuality in a healthy and informed manner. The aim of sexual health education is not only to provide knowledge about reproduction but also to promote responsible decision-making, healthy behaviors, and emotional well-being.

Key Components of Sexual Health Education:

1. **Anatomy and Reproductive Health:** Understanding the anatomy of the reproductive system is fundamental to adolescent sexual health education. Young people need to learn about the male and female reproductive systems, the menstrual cycle, sperm and egg production, and how conception occurs. Knowledge of fertility and the factors that influence reproductive health can empower adolescents to make informed choices regarding their health.

2. **Sexuality and Relationships:** Adolescents need to be educated about sexuality in a respectful and inclusive way. This includes understanding sexual orientation, gender identity, consent, and the emotional aspects of intimate relationships. Teaching adolescents about mutual respect, healthy boundaries, and communication skills is essential in fostering healthy relationships and preventing issues like sexual coercion, harassment, or assault.

3. **Contraception and Family Planning:** Educating adolescents about contraception is a critical part of sexual health education. Young people must understand the various forms of contraception available, including condoms, birth control pills, intrauterine devices (IUDs), and emergency contraception. Education about how these methods prevent pregnancy and protect against sexually transmitted infections (STIs) is essential for promoting safe sexual practices. It is important to emphasize that contraception is not only for preventing pregnancy but also for preventing the spread of STIs.

4. **Sexually Transmitted Infections (STIs) Prevention:** One of the most important aspects of adolescent sexual health education is informing young people about the risks of STIs and how they are transmitted. Emphasizing the importance of condom use, regular STI testing, and honest

communication with sexual partners is crucial in preventing the spread of infections like chlamydia, gonorrhea, and human papillomavirus (HPV). Adolescents should also be educated about the availability of vaccines, such as the HPV vaccine, which can protect against certain types of cancer and genital warts.

5. **Mental and Emotional Health:** Adolescence is a time of significant emotional development, and sexual health education should address mental health concerns related to puberty and sexual development. Topics like body image, self-esteem, and the emotional consequences of sexual activity should be discussed openly. Encouraging open dialogue and providing resources for support can help adolescents navigate the challenges they face as they develop their sexual identities.

Prevention: Empowering Adolescents with Knowledge

Prevention is at the heart of adolescent reproductive health. By providing adolescents with accurate information about puberty, sexual development, and reproductive health, we equip them to make healthy decisions that will benefit their physical, emotional, and social well-being.

1. **Preventing Early and Unintended Pregnancy:** One of the most pressing concerns in adolescent reproductive health is preventing early pregnancy. While many adolescents are capable of reproduction during puberty, they may not be emotionally or financially prepared to raise a child. Preventing early pregnancies through comprehensive sex education, access to contraception, and open communication can help young people delay parenthood until they are ready.

2. **Promoting Healthy Peer Relationships:** Peer pressure plays a significant role in adolescent decision-making, and navigating relationships can be challenging during these years. Teaching adolescents to form healthy, respectful relationships with peers can help prevent situations where they might feel pressured into engaging in sexual activity or risky behaviors. Additionally, fostering emotional intelligence and self-awareness can help adolescents recognize when a relationship is unhealthy or unsafe.

3. **Access to Healthcare Services:** Adolescents should have access to confidential and age-appropriate healthcare services, including reproductive health screenings, counseling, and STI testing. The availability of services like these ensures that young people can receive the care and support they need without fear of judgment or exposure. Healthcare providers should be trained to work with adolescents and provide guidance in a supportive and nonjudgmental manner.

4. **Engaging Parents and Caregivers:** Parents and caregivers play a pivotal role in adolescent reproductive health, and engaging them in conversations about puberty, sexual health, and prevention is essential. When adolescents feel comfortable talking to their parents or caregivers about these topics, they are more likely to make informed choices and seek help when necessary. Programs that offer training and support for parents can improve communication and reduce barriers to sexual health education.

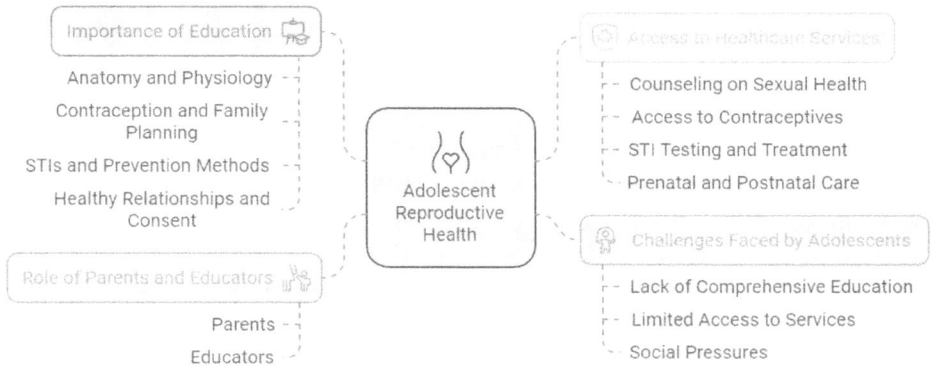

Conclusion

Adolescent reproductive health is foundational to long-term well-being, and investing in the education, prevention, and support of young people is essential to fostering healthy generations. Puberty, with its physical, emotional, and psychological changes, sets the stage for the rest of an individual's reproductive life. By equipping adolescents with the tools, they need to understand their bodies, make informed decisions, and navigate their sexual health with confidence, we empower them to lead healthy, fulfilling lives.

As society continues to evolve, so too should our approach to adolescent reproductive health. Emphasizing comprehensive, age-appropriate education, accessible healthcare, and open dialogue ensures that adolescents are supported throughout their journey toward sexual and reproductive maturity. With the right foundation, young people can enter adulthood prepared to make responsible, informed choices about their health, relationships, and futures.

Chapter 25

Reproductive Health in Your 20s and 30s

Introduction: The Foundation of Reproductive Health in Adulthood

Your 20s and 30s represent a crucial period in your reproductive life, laying the groundwork for both your present and future health. During these decades, many individuals experience significant life changes, such as pursuing higher education, starting careers, building relationships, and making important decisions about family planning. These years are often marked by fertility considerations, decisions about having children, and a growing awareness of sexual health.

Reproductive health in your 20s and 30s involves understanding your body's natural rhythms, making informed choices about contraception, preparing for potential pregnancies, and staying proactive about the prevention of sexually transmitted infections (STIs). It's also an ideal time to start cultivating habits that promote long-term reproductive wellness, including maintaining a healthy lifestyle, seeking regular medical check-ups, and addressing any concerns promptly.

This chapter delves into the reproductive health topics most relevant to individuals in their 20s and 30s, including fertility considerations, family planning options, and STI prevention strategies. By understanding the physiological changes that occur during these decades and making informed choices, individuals can protect their reproductive health and set the stage for a healthy future.

Fertility Considerations During Early Adulthood

Fertility is a major aspect of reproductive health in your 20s and 30s. This is the time when many individuals begin to actively consider their fertility, whether they are planning to start a family or exploring other options. However, it's important to recognize that fertility can vary significantly from person to person. Understanding how fertility works, how it changes over time, and when to seek help is crucial in making informed decisions about reproductive health.

Fertility in Your 20s: Peak Reproductive Years

For most people assigned female at birth, the 20s are considered the peak fertility years. During this time, fertility is typically at its highest, and the chances of conceiving are most favorable. However, even within this age range, many factors can influence fertility, including lifestyle choices, overall health, and environmental factors.

1. **Ovulation and Menstrual Cycle:** In your 20s, the menstrual cycle is often regular, with ovulation occurring around the middle of the cycle. Ovulation is the release of an egg from the ovary, and it is a critical component of fertility. If you are trying to conceive, understanding when ovulation occurs and tracking your menstrual cycle can help improve your chances of getting pregnant.

2. **Fertility Preservation:** While fertility is at its peak in your 20s, some people may face health conditions or life circumstances that make pregnancy less feasible in the future. For instance, individuals diagnosed with cancer may choose to freeze their eggs or embryos before undergoing treatments like chemotherapy that can affect fertility. In such cases, fertility preservation is an important option to consider.

3. **Contraception and Family Planning:** If you are not ready to have children in your 20s, contraception is an essential tool for preventing unintended pregnancies. From oral contraceptives (birth control pills) to long-acting

reversible contraceptives (LARCs) like IUDs and implants, there are many effective options to suit individual preferences and lifestyles.

It's also important to consider that some forms of contraception may affect fertility in the short term. For example, using birth control pills can take several months for the body to return to its natural hormonal state after discontinuation. However, most people will regain fertility relatively quickly after stopping hormonal contraception, especially in their 20s.

4. **Lifestyle Factors That Affect Fertility:** Your lifestyle choices during your 20s can significantly impact your fertility. Factors such as diet, exercise, alcohol consumption, smoking, and stress levels can all influence your reproductive health. For example, smoking is known to negatively affect egg quality, while excessive alcohol use and poor diet can decrease overall fertility. It is important to adopt healthy habits during this time, as they will not only benefit your reproductive health but also your overall well-being.

5. **STI Prevention and Fertility:** Preventing sexually transmitted infections (STIs) is essential in your 20s, as untreated STIs can cause long-term fertility issues. Conditions like chlamydia, gonorrhea, and human papillomavirus (HPV) can lead to complications such as pelvic inflammatory disease (PID), scarring of the fallopian tubes, and infertility. Using condoms, getting regular STI screenings, and communicating openly with sexual partners can help prevent STIs and protect your fertility.

Fertility in Your 30s: Preparing for Changes

While fertility is still good during your 30s, it gradually begins to decline, particularly after the age of 35. For individuals assigned female at birth, the number and quality of eggs begin to decrease, and the chances of getting pregnant naturally may begin to decline. However, many people in their 30s still experience healthy pregnancies and successful births, especially when they are aware of the changes and take proactive steps.

1. **Egg Quantity and Quality:** In your early 30s, the number of eggs in your ovaries starts to decline, and the quality of eggs may also begin to decrease. This means that even though ovulation still occurs, there may be fewer eggs to fertilize, and the chances of chromosomal abnormalities increase with age. This can lead to difficulties in conceiving, especially as you approach your mid-30s.

For some individuals, the decline in fertility may be subtle and not immediately noticeable. However, if pregnancy is taking longer than expected, it's a good idea to seek guidance from a healthcare provider. Tests like ovarian reserve testing, which measures hormone levels and egg quantity, can help assess fertility potential and guide future decisions.

2. **Fertility Treatments:** If conception is challenging, assisted reproductive technologies (ART), such as in vitro fertilization (IVF), may be an option. IVF involves extracting eggs from the ovaries, fertilizing them outside the body, and implanting the embryo in the uterus. This treatment has a higher success rate for women under 35 but can still be an option for those in their late 30s. Other fertility treatments may include intrauterine insemination (IUI), which involves placing sperm directly into the uterus.

3. **Lifestyle Adjustments for Better Fertility:** As you enter your 30s, it's even more important to focus on lifestyle factors that support fertility. Eating a balanced diet, exercising regularly, managing stress, and avoiding harmful substances like tobacco and excessive alcohol can help improve fertility and

increase your chances of conception. For instance, maintaining a healthy body weight is critical, as being overweight or underweight can impact ovulation and fertility.

4. **Prenatal Health and Screening:** As you reach your 30s, prenatal health becomes even more important. If you are considering pregnancy, taking steps to ensure a healthy pregnancy, such as taking prenatal vitamins with folic acid, is crucial. Additionally, it's recommended to have screenings for genetic conditions, such as Down syndrome, as the risk of chromosomal abnormalities increases with maternal age.

Regular check-ups with a gynecologist or obstetrician are also important to monitor overall reproductive health and discuss any concerns you may have. Conditions like polycystic ovary syndrome (PCOS), endometriosis, and fibroids may be more prevalent in your 30s and can affect fertility, so being aware of the signs and seeking medical advice can help manage these conditions.

5. **Fertility Preservation:** If you are unsure about having children in your 30s but want to preserve the option in the future, fertility preservation through egg freezing is a viable option. Egg freezing allows you to store healthy eggs for later use, which can be beneficial if you wish to delay pregnancy for personal or professional reasons.

Family Planning and Prevention of STIs in Your 20s and 30s

Family planning in your 20s and 30s is an important decision that involves determining when and how you would like to have children. This process can involve several factors, such as career goals, relationships, financial stability, and personal desires.

1. **Contraceptive Options:** There is a wide range of contraceptive methods available to help individuals in their 20s and 30s prevent unintended pregnancies. These methods include hormonal contraception (birth control pills, patches, injections, and implants), barrier methods (condoms and diaphragms), and permanent solutions like sterilization. It's important to choose a method that aligns with your lifestyle and health needs, and to review contraceptive options with a healthcare provider to find the best fit.
2. **STI Prevention:** In your 20s and 30s, it's vital to take measures to prevent the spread of STIs. Using condoms consistently and correctly during sexual activity is one of the most effective ways to protect against most STIs. Regular STI screenings, especially if you have new sexual partners or engage in high-risk behaviors, are essential for early detection and treatment.

Being informed about the available vaccines, such as the HPV vaccine, can also protect against certain strains of the virus that can lead to genital warts and cervical cancer.

3. **Communication and Shared Responsibility:** Family planning and STI prevention should be shared responsibilities between partners. Open communication about contraception, sexual health, and STI testing is crucial for ensuring a healthy, fulfilling sexual relationship. Discussing reproductive goals and preferences with a partner can help ensure that both parties are on the same page and ready to take proactive steps in managing reproductive health.

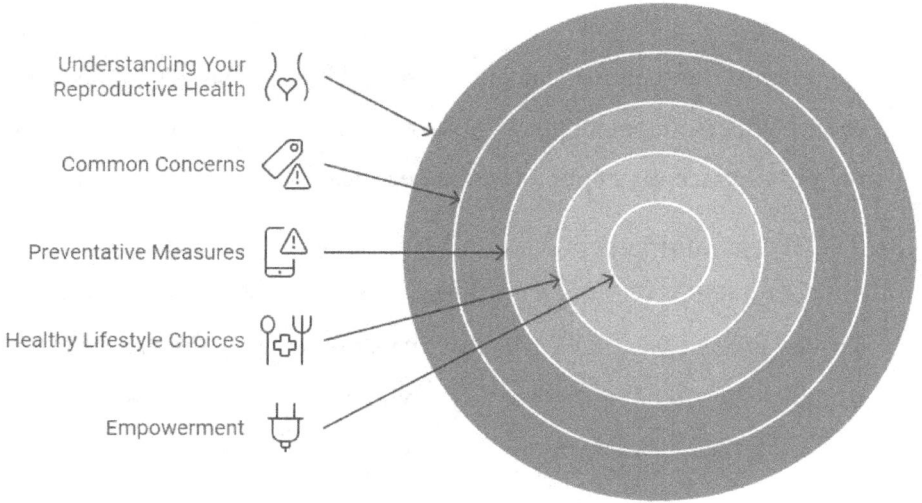

Conclusion

Prioritizing Reproductive Health in Your 20s and 30s

The decisions you make regarding reproductive health in your 20s and 30s will have a significant impact on your overall well-being and future reproductive outcomes. By understanding how fertility changes during these years, practicing safe sex, and making informed choices about contraception and family planning, you can set a strong foundation for a healthy reproductive future.

It's essential to stay proactive, communicate openly with healthcare providers, and be aware of how lifestyle choices affect fertility. This is a time of growth and opportunity, and with the right knowledge and support, you can confidently navigate the challenges and rewards of reproductive health during your 20s and 30s.

Chapter 26

Reproductive Health in Your 40s and Beyond

Introduction: The Evolution of Reproductive Health in Your 40s and Beyond

As you enter your 40s and beyond, your reproductive health undergoes significant changes. For many, this decade marks the transition from fertility to the end of reproductive years, accompanied by a range of physical, hormonal, and emotional changes. While it can be a time of reflection and adjustment, understanding the physiological shifts that occur, as well as how to manage them, empowers individuals to maintain good reproductive health, prevent potential complications, and adapt to this new phase of life with confidence.

During this stage, most people experience perimenopause, the period leading up to menopause, and ultimately, menopause itself. These changes are natural, but they often come with challenges, such as irregular menstrual cycles, hot flashes, mood swings, and more. Additionally, fertility becomes less predictable, and while pregnancy is still possible for some, the risks associated with conception and pregnancy increase after age 40. This chapter will explore how reproductive health evolves during this time, the management of menopause and perimenopause, and the risks and considerations regarding fertility and pregnancy in your 40s and beyond.

Managing Menopause and Perimenopause

Menopause is a natural part of aging that signals the end of the menstrual cycle and reproductive capability. It is diagnosed after 12 consecutive months without menstruation, typically occurring between the ages of 45 and 55, although the timing can vary. Perimenopause is the transitional phase leading up to menopause, during which the body begins to experience hormonal fluctuations. These changes can lead to various symptoms that may affect your overall well-being.

Understanding Perimenopause

Perimenopause can begin several years before menopause, usually in a person's late 30s to early 40s. It is characterized by irregular menstrual cycles and fluctuating hormone levels, particularly estrogen and progesterone. These hormonal changes can have a wide range of effects, including changes in menstrual patterns, hot flashes, night sweats, vaginal dryness, sleep disturbances, mood swings, and reduced fertility.

1. **Irregular Periods and Hormonal Fluctuations:** During perimenopause, your periods may become irregular, occurring more frequently or skipping months. These changes in menstrual patterns can be frustrating, but they are a normal part of the process. The decrease in progesterone and estrogen levels during this time can lead to shorter or longer cycles, lighter or heavier bleeding, and more frequent spotting. Some individuals may experience heavier periods during perimenopause, while others may have lighter flows.

2. **Hot Flashes and Night Sweats:** One of the hallmark symptoms of perimenopause and menopause is the hot flash. These sudden feelings of intense warmth or heat, often accompanied by sweating and redness, are caused by the body's fluctuating estrogen levels. Hot flashes can occur throughout the day or night, and when they happen during sleep, they are known as night sweats. While hot flashes can be bothersome, there are various treatment options available to help manage them, such as hormone

replacement therapy (HRT), lifestyle changes, and natural remedies like herbal supplements.

3. **Vaginal Dryness and Decreased Libido:** As estrogen levels decline during perimenopause and menopause, many individuals experience vaginal dryness, which can lead to discomfort during intercourse. Vaginal dryness is often accompanied by a thinning of the vaginal walls, which can make the tissue more fragile and susceptible to irritation. Additionally, changes in libido may occur, which is also influenced by hormonal shifts, age-related changes in sexual function, and emotional factors. Vaginal moisturizers, lubricants, and hormone therapies can help alleviate dryness, while communication with a partner and counseling can address any emotional or psychological concerns related to libido changes.

4. **Mood Swings and Mental Health:** Mood swings, irritability, and even anxiety or depression are common during perimenopause. These emotional changes can be caused by hormonal fluctuations, but they may also be influenced by lifestyle, stress, and underlying mental health conditions. Women may feel more emotional or experience difficulty with concentration or memory, often referred to as "brain fog." Regular physical activity, stress reduction techniques, and counseling or therapy can be beneficial in managing mood changes during this time.

5. **Sleep Disturbances:** Hormonal changes during perimenopause and menopause can interfere with sleep. Many individuals experience difficulty falling asleep, staying asleep, or waking up feeling unrested. The combination of hot flashes, night sweats, and hormonal imbalances can make it harder to maintain healthy sleep patterns. Addressing these sleep

issues through lifestyle changes, good sleep hygiene, and sometimes medication can help improve the quality of sleep during this time.

Navigating Menopause

Menopause, defined as the cessation of menstruation for 12 consecutive months, typically occurs around age 51, although it can happen earlier or later. The transition to menopause brings about more permanent changes to reproductive health, including the end of menstruation and fertility. The symptoms associated with menopause often persist for several years but may eventually subside as the body adjusts to lower hormone levels.

1. **Hormonal Changes and the End of Fertility:** Menopause marks the permanent cessation of ovulation and menstruation. As the ovaries produce less estrogen and progesterone, menstruation stops, and the ability to conceive naturally ceases. For many, menopause brings a sense of relief from the monthly cycle, but it can also lead to emotional challenges and concerns about aging and the end of fertility. For some, the transition to menopause can be a time of rediscovery and self-reflection, while others may experience feelings of loss or frustration about not being able to have children.

2. **Hormone Replacement Therapy (HRT):** Hormone replacement therapy (HRT) is a common treatment option for managing menopausal symptoms. It involves taking synthetic hormones to replace the estrogen and progesterone that the body no longer produces. HRT can alleviate symptoms like hot flashes, night sweats, vaginal dryness, and mood changes. However, it is important to discuss the risks and benefits of HRT with a healthcare provider, as it may not be suitable for everyone. For those who cannot take

HRT, other medications, including selective serotonin reuptake inhibitors (SSRIs) and non-hormonal treatments, can help manage symptoms.

3. **Lifestyle Adjustments and Self-Care:** Embracing a healthy lifestyle is crucial during menopause. Eating a balanced diet rich in calcium and vitamin D, engaging in regular physical activity, and avoiding smoking can help mitigate some of the health risks associated with menopause, such as osteoporosis and cardiovascular disease. Weight management, stress reduction, and getting enough sleep are also key factors in improving overall health and well-being during menopause.

Fertility After Age 40 and Risks During Pregnancy

Fertility naturally declines as you age, with more significant changes occurring after the age of 35. While conception is still possible in your 40s, it becomes increasingly difficult due to the decrease in both the quantity and quality of eggs. This chapter explores the complexities of fertility and pregnancy after age 40, as well as the associated risks and considerations.

Declining Fertility After 40

As individuals approach their 40s, the body's ability to produce eggs with normal chromosomal makeup decreases. This can result in a reduced chance of conception and an increased risk of miscarriage. Additionally, ovulation may become less predictable, and cycles may become more irregular. While many individuals in their 40s still conceive naturally, the chances of pregnancy decrease significantly with age. For example, the fertility rate for a 40-year-old is about 5 percent per cycle, compared to about 20 percent for a 30-year-old.

1. **Ovarian Reserve and Egg Quality:** Ovarian reserve refers to the quantity and quality of eggs in the ovaries. By the age of 40, most individuals have a

significantly reduced ovarian reserve, and the remaining eggs may be of lower quality. This means that even if ovulation occurs, the chances of producing a healthy egg that can be fertilized are reduced. To assess ovarian reserve, healthcare providers can conduct tests such as an ultrasound to check the ovaries or blood tests to measure hormone levels (e.g., AMH, FSH, and estradiol).

2. **Assisted Reproductive Technologies (ART):** For those over 40 who want to conceive, assisted reproductive technologies (ART), including in vitro fertilization (IVF), may offer a solution. ART procedures like IVF allow eggs to be fertilized outside the body, and the embryos are implanted into the uterus. IVF success rates are lower for individuals over 40, and often, egg donors are used to improve the chances of success. However, ART can still be an option for those seeking pregnancy later in life.

Risks of Pregnancy After 40

Pregnancy after 40 comes with an increased risk of complications for both the mother and the baby. It's essential to be aware of these risks and seek appropriate care and monitoring throughout the pregnancy.

1. **Increased Risk of Chromosomal Abnormalities:** As maternal age increases, the risk of chromosomal abnormalities, such as Down syndrome, increases. Prenatal testing, including non-invasive prenatal testing (NIPT) and amniocentesis, can assess the risk of genetic conditions. Discussing these tests with a healthcare provider is important for making informed decisions.

2. **Gestational Diabetes and Hypertension:** Pregnant individuals over 40 are at an increased risk for gestational diabetes and hypertension (high blood

pressure during pregnancy). These conditions can affect both the health of the mother and the baby. Regular prenatal visits and monitoring are crucial for managing these risks and ensuring the best possible outcomes.

3. **Miscarriage and Preterm Birth:** The risk of miscarriage increases with age, especially after 40. Additionally, there is an elevated risk of preterm birth (birth before 37 weeks) and low birth weight. Advanced maternal age may also increase the likelihood of requiring a cesarean section due to complications such as fetal distress or abnormal positioning.

4. **Emotional and Psychological Considerations:** Pregnancy at an older age can be emotionally and mentally challenging. Some individuals may feel anxiety about their ability to carry the pregnancy to term or concerns about parenting at an older age. Counseling, support groups, and open communication with a partner or healthcare provider can help manage these feelings and provide emotional support.

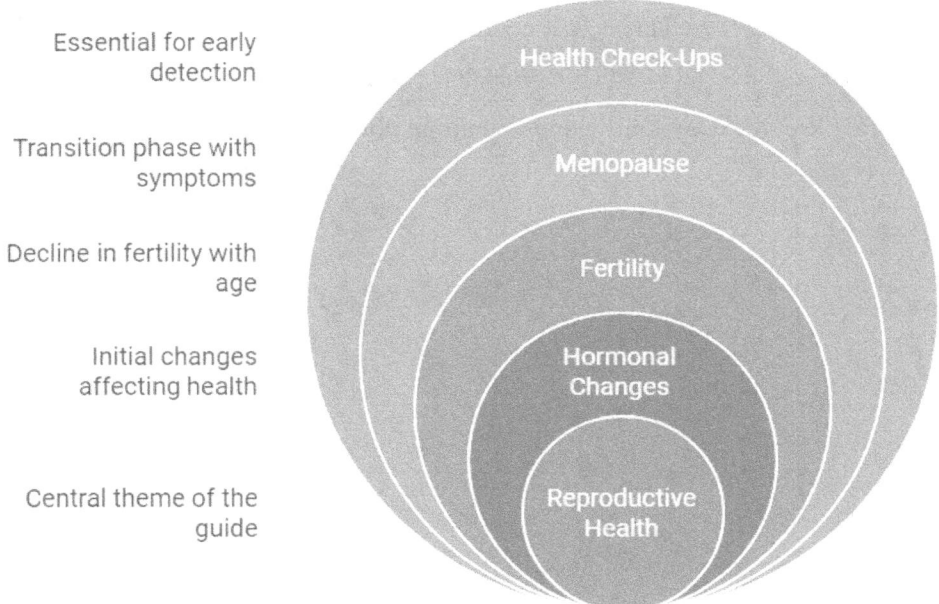

Conclusion

Reproductive health in your 40s and beyond is a dynamic and evolving process. While fertility naturally declines with age, there are still many ways to manage reproductive health and make informed decisions about family planning and pregnancy. By understanding the physical changes that come with perimenopause, menopause, and aging, you can adopt a proactive approach to maintain overall health, manage symptoms, and address any concerns about fertility or pregnancy.

Fertility preservation, assisted reproductive technologies, and a focus on overall wellness, including lifestyle changes and mental health support, can empower individuals in their 40s to navigate this phase with confidence and clarity. Embracing the changes that come with age, while also prioritizing your reproductive and overall health, ensures that you can continue to live a fulfilling and vibrant life, regardless of where you are in your reproductive journey.

Chapter 27

The Role of Partners in Reproductive Health

Introduction: Reproductive Health as a Shared Journey

Reproductive health is not just an individual concern; it is a shared journey for couples navigating challenges, decisions, and health issues together. Whether dealing with infertility, sexually transmitted infections (STIs), menstrual health issues, or other reproductive challenges, the role of partners in supporting one another is crucial for emotional, physical, and psychological well-being. The dynamics of reproductive health issues are complex, and understanding how to navigate them as a team can strengthen relationships, provide much-needed support, and improve the chances of successful outcomes.

This chapter will explore the importance of mutual support in reproductive health, how couples can address challenges such as infertility and STIs, and the role of emotional connection and communication in managing these difficulties. It will also discuss practical ways to ensure that both partners are involved and supportive throughout the process.

The Importance of Emotional Support

Reproductive health issues can be emotionally taxing for both partners. The impact of dealing with health conditions like infertility, hormone imbalances, or an STI can strain relationships if not managed properly. For individuals experiencing these challenges, the emotional burden can include feelings of frustration, inadequacy, guilt, or isolation. For the partner, the situation may also lead to feelings of helplessness or confusion.

The emotional support of a partner can alleviate much of this stress. Compassionate communication, mutual understanding, and patience are key elements in providing emotional security and fostering resilience as a couple. A strong partnership that is based on empathy and openness is better equipped to navigate the highs and lows of reproductive health challenges.

Managing Infertility as a Team

Infertility affects approximately 10-15% of couples worldwide. It can be a profound source of stress, sadness, and frustration for both partners, as it challenges the shared vision of starting or expanding a family. However, infertility should never be viewed as the problem of one partner; it is a joint issue that requires mutual support and shared responsibility.

1. **Understanding and Communication:** One of the first steps in addressing infertility as a couple is to engage in open and honest communication. Discussing feelings, fears, and expectations is critical to preventing misunderstandings. Partners may have different emotional reactions to infertility, and acknowledging these differences without judgment can help build a supportive foundation. By understanding each other's perspectives, couples can ensure that both partners feel heard and valued.

2. **Exploring Treatment Options Together:** Couples should explore treatment options together and make joint decisions. Assisted reproductive technologies (ART), such as in vitro fertilization (IVF), intrauterine insemination (IUI), or fertility preservation (e.g., egg/sperm freezing), are common choices for couples struggling with infertility. These procedures can be physically and emotionally draining, and it is essential that both partners are actively involved in the decision-making process. When partners work as a team in exploring treatments, they are more likely to feel empowered and united in their efforts to conceive.

3. **Supporting Each Other During Treatments:** Fertility treatments often require numerous appointments, injections, tests, and even surgeries. During these times, one partner may need more physical or emotional support than the other. It is important that both partners recognize the physical and psychological strain of the process and remain flexible and supportive. Simple gestures like attending appointments together, being a listening ear, and offering encouragement can help ease anxiety and create a sense of partnership and solidarity.

4. **Coping with Setbacks and Loss:** Not all fertility treatments result in success, and many couples experience miscarriage or failed cycles, which can lead to intense grief. The emotional pain of losing a pregnancy, or failing to conceive after multiple attempts, is felt by both partners, even if it manifests differently. A couple's ability to cope with setbacks together can significantly impact their healing process. By acknowledging and validating each other's grief, partners can form a stronger emotional bond and find ways to move forward.

Addressing STIs as a Team

Sexually transmitted infections (STIs) can affect anyone who is sexually active, and when one partner is diagnosed with an STI, it is important that both partners approach the situation collaboratively and respectfully. STIs such as genital herpes, gonorrhea, chlamydia, and HIV can have significant implications for reproductive health, and addressing them together is vital for ensuring both partners' well-being.

1. **Honest Communication:** Open communication is crucial when one or both partners are diagnosed with an STI. Discussing the situation honestly,

without fear of judgment or blame, helps reduce the emotional burden. Both partners should share their feelings, concerns, and any questions they may have about their diagnosis and treatment options. It's essential that both partners understand the potential risks, transmission routes, and prevention methods to ensure that their sexual health remains a shared responsibility.

2. **Seeking Medical Advice Together:** When one partner is diagnosed with an STI, the other partner should seek medical advice, even if they have not shown symptoms. This allows both partners to get tested, receive treatment if necessary, and prevent reinfection. Couples should also educate themselves on STI prevention methods, such as using condoms, regular testing, and safe sexual practices. Working together to make informed decisions about sexual health and maintaining a proactive approach to prevention helps reduce the emotional and physical consequences of STIs.

3. **Managing the Psychological Impact of STIs:** An STI diagnosis can lead to feelings of shame, guilt, or embarrassment, and these emotions can affect the couple's relationship. It is important for both partners to approach the situation without blame and with a focus on healing. Counseling or therapy can help partners cope with the emotional impact of an STI diagnosis, providing tools to communicate more effectively and support each other through the recovery process. Offering emotional reassurance, expressing care, and reinforcing commitment to one another can strengthen the bond in times of uncertainty.

Joint Decisions Regarding Birth Control and Family Planning

Family planning is one of the most important decisions a couple can make, and it requires careful consideration of reproductive health, financial stability, and emotional readiness. Deciding whether or not to have children, when to have children, and how many children to have are significant decisions that should be made collaboratively. The partner's role in this decision-making process cannot be underestimated.

1. **Shared Responsibility in Contraception:** Contraceptive choices should involve both partners in order to ensure that both individuals are comfortable with the methods chosen. Birth control options range from hormonal methods (e.g., the pill, implants) to barrier methods (e.g., condoms) and permanent options (e.g., sterilization). Discussing the pros and cons of each option, as well as considering personal preferences, lifestyle, and health factors, allows couples to make informed choices about contraception together.

2. **Planning for Parenthood:** For couples who are ready to start a family, family planning discussions are vital. This involves not only deciding when to try for a child, but also considering financial, emotional, and health factors that may influence the timing of pregnancy. Preconception health checks, such as ensuring that both partners are in good physical health and addressing any existing reproductive health issues, can increase the likelihood of a successful pregnancy.

3. **Balancing Career and Parenthood:** Balancing professional and personal life when considering starting a family can be a challenging decision for many couples. The role of the partner in this conversation is essential, as both individuals must share the responsibilities of child-rearing and household duties. Open discussions about career goals, personal aspirations, and shared responsibilities can help mitigate stress and ensure that both partners are on the same page about family life.

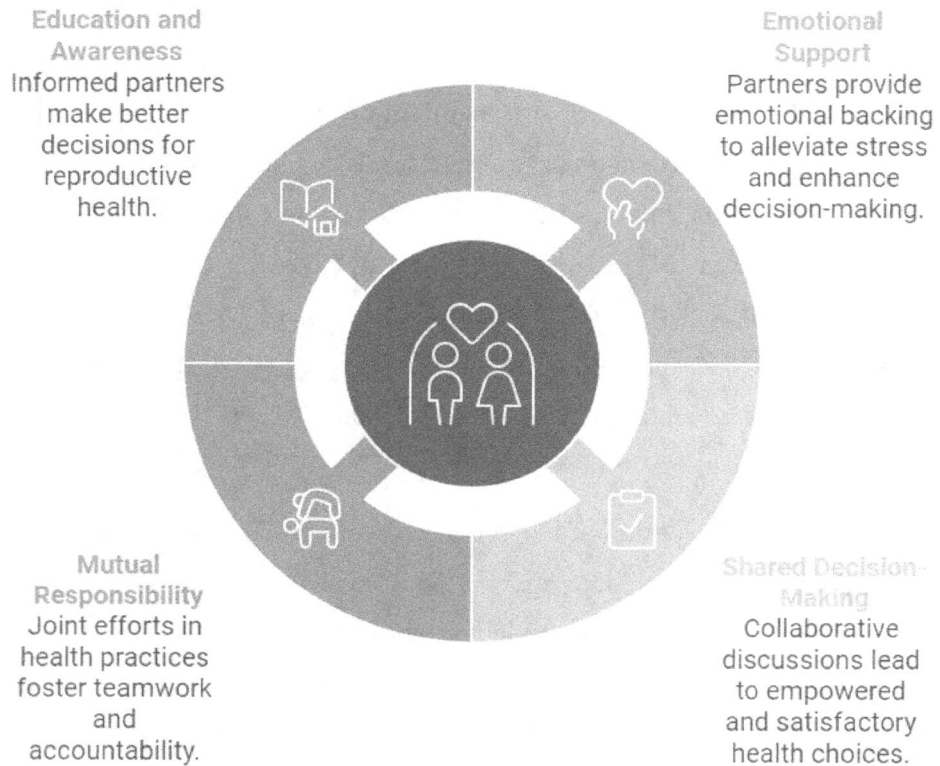

Partner Roles in Reproductive Health

Education and Awareness
Informed partners make better decisions for reproductive health.

Emotional Support
Partners provide emotional backing to alleviate stress and enhance decision-making.

Mutual Responsibility
Joint efforts in health practices foster teamwork and accountability.

Shared Decision-Making
Collaborative discussions lead to empowered and satisfactory health choices.

Conclusion

Navigating reproductive health challenges requires empathy, patience, and collaboration. Whether dealing with infertility, STIs, or making family planning decisions, the role of partners is essential in ensuring that both individuals feel supported and valued. Effective communication, emotional understanding, shared responsibility, and a focus on mutual respect can strengthen the relationship and help partners overcome challenges together.

The emotional and physical support of a partner can make a significant difference in the way individuals experience and manage reproductive health issues. By standing together as a team, couples can navigate these challenges with resilience and love, creating a foundation of trust and cooperation that will enhance their relationship and promote better reproductive health outcomes.

Chapter 28

Coping with Infertility: Emotional Support and Treatment

Introduction: The Emotional Journey of Infertility

Infertility is a deeply emotional and often overwhelming experience that affects millions of individuals and couples around the world. It is not just a medical condition; it is a profound life challenge that touches every aspect of a person's emotional and psychological well-being. The path to understanding and managing infertility involves not only physical treatments but also emotional resilience and coping strategies. Whether faced by an individual or a couple, the emotional journey of infertility can bring about a wide range of feelings, including sadness, frustration, anxiety, guilt, and a sense of inadequacy.

This chapter will explore the psychological and emotional impact of infertility, providing insights into how individuals can cope with these challenges. It will also discuss coping strategies, the role of emotional support, and the importance of seeking professional help. Navigating infertility is never easy, but with the right resources and mindset, individuals and couples can build the emotional strength needed to face the obstacles infertility presents.

Understanding the Emotional Impact of Infertility

Infertility is often thought of purely as a physical or medical issue, but its emotional toll can be just as significant, if not more so. The process of trying to conceive can evoke a range of emotions, especially when conception doesn't occur as expected. For many, infertility is associated with a profound sense of loss and grief, as it disrupts the vision of starting or growing a family. These emotional reactions can be both immediate and long-term, and it's crucial to understand that they are a normal part of the infertility experience.

1. **Feelings of Grief and Loss:** The grief associated with infertility is often compared to the mourning process after a death. People may experience denial, anger, bargaining, depression, and acceptance as they come to terms with the reality of their infertility. The loss of the idealized version of family life, the disappointment of failed attempts, and the uncertainty of what the future holds can weigh heavily on one's emotional health. Understanding that these feelings are normal is a first step in coping.

2. **Frustration and Isolation:** One of the most challenging aspects of infertility is the feeling of being out of control. The inability to conceive despite trying or seeking medical intervention can lead to frustration and hopelessness. Additionally, many individuals undergoing infertility treatment may feel isolated, as the topic can be difficult to discuss openly with family, friends, or even partners. Society's expectations regarding family life often add pressure to the emotional burden of infertility, making those affected feel as though they are failing in some way.

3. **Guilt and Blame:** Individuals and couples often experience feelings of guilt, particularly if they perceive themselves as responsible for their infertility. Women, in particular, may internalize the blame, as infertility is often viewed as a woman's issue, even though both men and women can be affected. Men may also experience guilt or feel emasculated, especially if their infertility diagnosis comes from issues related to sperm quality or count. The weight of guilt can be debilitating and prevent individuals from fully processing their emotions or seeking the support they need.

4. **Anxiety and Uncertainty:** The uncertainty surrounding infertility can create ongoing anxiety. Individuals may find themselves constantly wondering about their chances of conception, the effectiveness of treatments, or the

future of their reproductive health. Anxiety can be heightened by the unpredictability of fertility treatments, such as in vitro fertilization (IVF), where success rates are never guaranteed. The emotional rollercoaster of starting treatment, undergoing cycles, and facing potential failure can lead to stress, insomnia, and persistent worry.

Coping Strategies for Managing Infertility-Related Emotions

Coping with infertility requires a multi-faceted approach that involves addressing emotional, psychological, and physical needs. While it is important to acknowledge the pain and frustration of infertility, developing coping strategies can help individuals and couples manage their emotions and maintain their mental health throughout the process. Here are some effective coping strategies for those facing infertility:

1. **Allowing Yourself to Grieve:** It is essential to acknowledge and honor the grief associated with infertility. Suppressing emotions or pretending that everything is fine can exacerbate feelings of isolation and anxiety. Giving yourself permission to grieve and experiencing those emotions fully is an important step in moving forward. This might include crying, talking about your feelings, or taking time away from fertility treatments to reflect and process the situation. Grief is not linear, and it may resurface at unexpected times, but it is a normal part of the healing process.

2. **Open Communication with Your Partner:** Infertility is often experienced as a couple's issue, and the emotional burden can be shared. Open, honest communication with your partner is critical in coping with the stress and disappointment that infertility brings. Talking openly about fears, frustrations, and desires for the future fosters understanding and helps

prevent emotional distance between partners. It is also important to recognize that both partners may process infertility differently. Respecting these differences while maintaining open dialogue can strengthen the relationship during challenging times.

3. **Seeking Support from Loved Ones:** While infertility can feel isolating, there is often comfort in knowing that friends and family care and want to offer support. However, not everyone will understand what it's like to experience infertility, and conversations can sometimes feel uncomfortable or inadequate. It's important to communicate with friends and family about your needs and boundaries. Let them know how they can best support you, whether by simply listening or offering a distraction. Sometimes, sharing your emotions with others who are supportive can help alleviate the emotional burden.

4. **Joining Support Groups:** Connecting with others who are going through similar experiences can be incredibly helpful. Support groups, whether in-person or online, provide a safe and non-judgmental space for sharing struggles, venting frustrations, and offering advice. Being part of a group allows individuals to feel less isolated and helps build a sense of community. It also offers the opportunity to hear others' coping strategies and successes, providing hope for those currently undergoing treatments.

5. **Mindfulness and Relaxation Techniques:** The emotional strain of infertility can be overwhelming, but mindfulness and relaxation practices can help reduce stress and promote emotional well-being. Techniques such as meditation, deep breathing exercises, yoga, and progressive muscle relaxation can be particularly helpful in managing anxiety and depression. Mindfulness encourages individuals to stay present in the moment, rather

than becoming overwhelmed by the uncertainty of the future. These practices can promote relaxation, improve sleep, and reduce the overall emotional burden of infertility.

6. **Journaling and Creative Expression:** Writing about your emotions, fears, and hopes can serve as a form of emotional release. Journaling allows individuals to reflect on their journey, express difficult emotions, and track their progress. It can also provide a sense of control in an otherwise unpredictable process. Creative expression, such as drawing, painting, or even crafting, can serve as an outlet for emotions and provide a therapeutic distraction from the stress of fertility treatments.

Seeking Professional Help

While self-care strategies and support from friends and family can be invaluable, professional help can play a critical role in managing the emotional toll of infertility. A mental health professional, particularly one experienced in reproductive health, can offer specialized support to help individuals and couples cope with infertility.

1. **Therapy and Counseling:** Therapy provides a safe, confidential space where individuals can talk about their emotional challenges without fear of judgment. Cognitive-behavioral therapy (CBT) is often used to help people reframe negative thoughts and manage anxiety related to infertility. Couples counseling can also help partners navigate relationship challenges, improve communication, and address emotional concerns related to fertility treatments. Many therapists also offer support for grief and loss, which can be particularly useful when experiencing miscarriages or failed cycles.

2. **Fertility Coaches:** Fertility coaches are trained professionals who specialize in supporting individuals through the fertility process. They offer practical guidance, emotional support, and motivation during fertility treatments, and they can help individuals develop healthy coping strategies. Fertility coaching focuses on empowering individuals and couples to make informed decisions while navigating the emotional rollercoaster of infertility.

3. **Psychiatric Support:** For those who may be struggling with severe anxiety, depression, or feelings of hopelessness, psychiatric intervention may be necessary. Medications such as antidepressants or anti-anxiety medications may be prescribed to help individuals manage their emotional health. It's important to discuss potential treatments with a psychiatrist who specializes in reproductive health, as some medications may affect fertility.

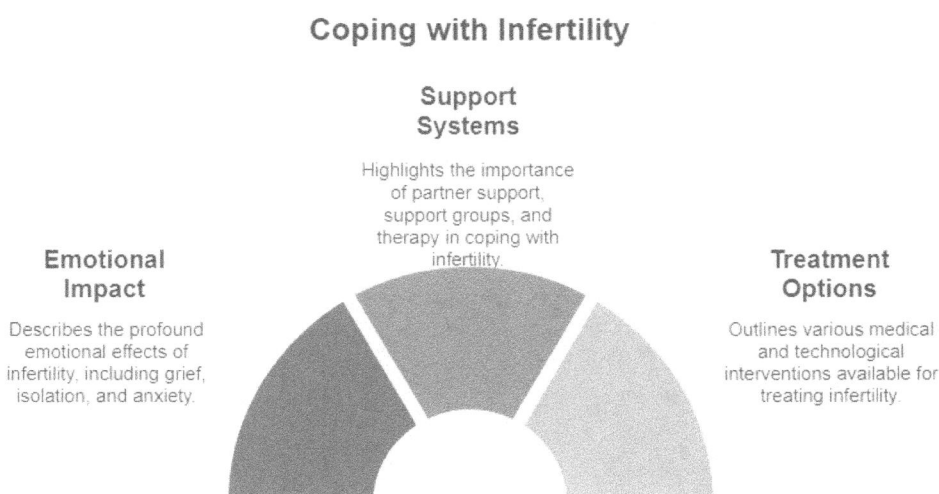

Conclusion

Infertility is undeniably a challenging and emotionally charged experience, but with the right support and coping strategies, individuals and couples can navigate its ups and downs with resilience and hope. Recognizing the emotional impact, developing healthy coping mechanisms, seeking professional help when necessary, and maintaining open communication with loved ones are all essential elements in managing the emotional journey of infertility. Though the road may be long and difficult, many couples eventually find their way toward their desired outcome—whether through successful conception, adoption, or alternative paths to parenthood.

Ultimately, infertility is not just about the medical treatments; it is about the emotional strength and support those individuals and couples draw upon to face the challenge. With resilience, hope, and the right resources, couples can emerge from the experience stronger and more united, ready to embrace their future with confidence and compassion.

Chapter 29

Managing the Diagnosis of Reproductive Cancers

Introduction: The Emotional Toll of Reproductive Cancer Diagnoses

Receiving a diagnosis of reproductive cancer—whether it involves the uterus, ovaries, cervix, prostate, or testes—can be a life-altering moment. It not only affects an individual's physical health but also profoundly impacts their emotional, psychological, and social well-being. The shock, fear, and uncertainty that accompany a cancer diagnosis can be overwhelming, and coping with this reality is often more challenging than the physical treatment itself.

Reproductive cancers can affect anyone, regardless of gender, age, or background. Women may face uterine, ovarian, or cervical cancer, while men can be diagnosed with prostate cancer. All these cancers carry their own unique set of challenges, but one of the most significant aspects is how the diagnosis affects an individual's reproductive health. The fear of infertility, loss of fertility, sexual dysfunction, and changes in one's body can amplify the emotional burden of cancer. In addition to the physical toll, there are deep emotional struggles with the uncertainty of treatment outcomes, the future of one's health, and the potential impact on intimate relationships.

This chapter will explore how individuals can manage the emotional and psychological toll of reproductive cancer diagnoses, the crucial role of support groups, and how therapy can assist in the journey toward healing. Understanding that these emotional reactions are a natural part of the cancer experience and knowing how to navigate them can significantly improve quality of life during and after treatment.

The Initial Shock and Emotional Response

The emotional response to a reproductive cancer diagnosis can be immediate and intense. Each person's reaction is unique, but common emotional responses often include shock, disbelief, fear, and sadness. The news of cancer can feel like an overwhelming burden, and many individuals may struggle to comprehend the reality of their diagnosis. Here are some common emotional stages individuals may experience:

1. **Shock and Denial:** Upon first hearing the diagnosis, many individuals may experience a sense of numbness or disbelief. It is difficult to accept that cancer is affecting the reproductive system, and often people may deny or minimize the situation as a defense mechanism. This initial response can last for hours, days, or weeks, depending on how the diagnosis is received and the person's ability to process the information. Denial is a way for the mind to protect itself from overwhelming distress, and while it is a natural response, it is important to eventually face the reality of the diagnosis to begin emotional healing.

2. **Fear and Anxiety:** Fear is a prominent emotional response to reproductive cancer. Individuals fear the unknown—about the cancer's prognosis, the side effects of treatment, and the possibility of infertility or changes in sexuality. The fear of death and uncertainty about the future can also lead to heightened anxiety. It is essential to acknowledge these fears and manage them, rather than letting them overwhelm daily life. Support systems, therapy, and coping mechanisms can help manage this fear, offering a sense of control and agency in an otherwise uncontrollable situation.

3. **Sadness and Grief:** A cancer diagnosis often brings feelings of sadness, especially when the individual is confronted with the potential for life-altering treatments. The idea of undergoing surgery, radiation, or

chemotherapy to treat cancer can be daunting, and for many, the fear of losing fertility, sexual function, or physical appearance is deeply saddening. The grief of losing one's former sense of self—whether that involves the loss of reproductive health or a part of one's body—is an incredibly valid emotional response. This grief can range from fleeting sadness to deep, persistent sorrow, but recognizing it is key to moving forward.

4. **Anger and Frustration:** It is not uncommon for individuals to feel angry after receiving a cancer diagnosis. They may be angry at their bodies for betraying them or angry at the unfairness of the situation. People may also feel frustration toward the healthcare system, family members, or even themselves for not being able to control or prevent the diagnosis. Anger is a healthy emotional response to injustice, but when it becomes chronic, it can interfere with treatment and emotional recovery. Finding healthy outlets for anger, such as therapy or physical activities, can help alleviate this frustration.

The Impact on Identity and Relationships

One of the most profound effects of a reproductive cancer diagnosis is the impact it can have on one's sense of identity. For individuals diagnosed with cancer affecting the reproductive system, the threat to their fertility or sexual health can lead to a crisis of identity. This is particularly significant for individuals who had hoped to have children or those who equate their reproductive health with their sense of femininity or masculinity. In some cases, the fear of losing these functions may feel like losing a key part of oneself.

1. **Fertility Concerns and Loss:** For women, reproductive cancers often raise concerns about the potential for infertility, especially with treatments such as

hysterectomy, chemotherapy, or radiation. Men diagnosed with prostate cancer may worry about erectile dysfunction or the ability to father children. Fertility preservation options, such as sperm or egg freezing, may be available before treatment, but for many, the possibility of infertility is a significant emotional burden.

2. **Sexual Health and Body Image:** The physical effects of cancer treatments, such as changes in appearance, energy levels, and sexual function, can affect self-esteem and body image. Surgery, radiation, and chemotherapy may leave visible scars or result in weight gain or loss. These physical changes can affect how individuals view themselves and how they feel about their attractiveness or desirability. For many, there is also the challenge of intimacy with partners. Sexual activity may be physically uncomfortable or emotionally challenging, and communication with a partner about these concerns is critical to maintaining a healthy relationship.

3. **Impact on Relationships:** A cancer diagnosis can put a significant strain on both romantic and familial relationships. Partners may experience stress, anxiety, and a desire to provide support, but may not always know how to do so. Couples may struggle with the emotional toll of the diagnosis and treatment, and it is important to navigate these challenges together. Open communication, patience, and mutual support can strengthen relationships during this difficult time.

The Role of Support Groups

Support groups offer a vital space for individuals facing reproductive cancer to share experiences, exchange advice, and provide emotional support. These groups allow individuals to connect with others who understand their struggles, providing comfort and reducing feelings of isolation. Support groups can be in-person or online and may focus on a particular type of cancer, gender-specific concerns, or general cancer support.

1. **Shared Experience and Comfort:** One of the greatest benefits of support groups is the opportunity to connect with others who are going through similar experiences. Knowing that others share the same fears, challenges, and triumphs can reduce feelings of isolation and loneliness. Support groups can offer a sense of community and solidarity, which is essential in managing the emotional journey of cancer.

2. **Emotional Expression and Healing:** Support groups create a safe space for individuals to express their emotions without judgment. Talking openly about feelings of fear, anger, sadness, and hope can promote emotional healing and provide clarity during uncertain times. Sharing experiences with others can also offer coping strategies that individuals may not have considered, helping them to process their emotions and navigate their treatment journey more effectively.

3. **Educational Resources:** Many support groups also provide education about reproductive cancer and its treatment. Learning about the medical aspects of the diagnosis from others who are further along in their journey can be reassuring. Support group members may share tips for managing side effects, post-treatment recovery, or fertility preservation, which can help individuals feel more informed and empowered.

The Role of Therapy in Managing Emotional Health

While support groups are beneficial, professional therapy plays a crucial role in managing the psychological impact of reproductive cancer. A licensed therapist or counselor can offer individualized care tailored to a person's unique emotional needs. Therapy provides a private and confidential environment where individuals can explore deep feelings of fear, grief, or anxiety. Cognitive-behavioral therapy (CBT) is a common therapeutic approach that helps individuals identify negative thought patterns and replace them with healthier, more balanced perspectives. CBT can be particularly effective in managing anxiety, depression, and stress during the cancer journey.

1. **Coping Mechanisms and Emotional Regulation:** Therapists can teach individuals coping mechanisms to handle the emotional stress of cancer treatment. Techniques such as mindfulness, relaxation exercises, and stress management tools can be taught to help individuals regulate their emotional responses to the situation. These techniques can also improve physical health by reducing the impact of stress on the body.

2. **Couples Therapy:** For couples facing reproductive cancer, therapy can help them address the unique challenges they face together. Couples therapy provides a space for both partners to express their feelings, concerns, and fears in a safe and guided environment. It also helps couples navigate complex topics like intimacy, communication, and future planning, which can be particularly challenging during cancer treatment.

3. **Grief Counseling:** Grief counseling can be particularly helpful for individuals facing reproductive cancer who are grieving the loss of fertility or sexual health. A therapist can help individuals process their grief and create healthy ways of coping with the loss. Through grief counseling, individuals can learn how to mourn while continuing to live their lives and find new hope for the future.

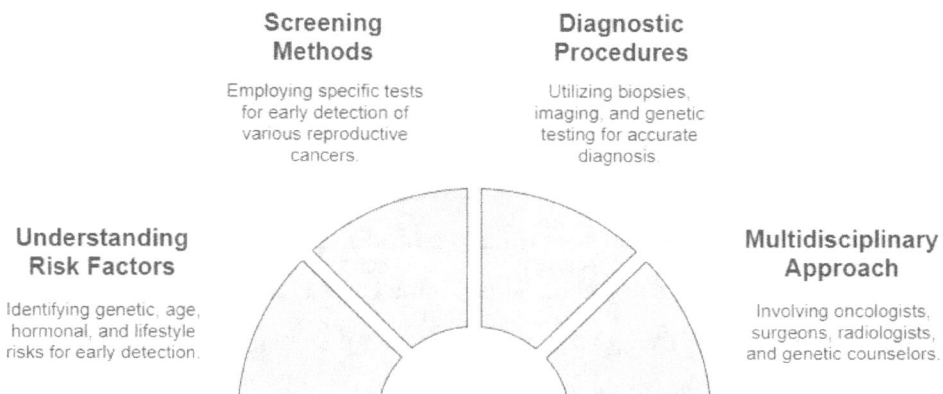

Managing the Diagnosis of Reproductive Cancers

- **Screening Methods**: Employing specific tests for early detection of various reproductive cancers.
- **Diagnostic Procedures**: Utilizing biopsies, imaging, and genetic testing for accurate diagnosis.
- **Understanding Risk Factors**: Identifying genetic, age, hormonal, and lifestyle risks for early detection.
- **Multidisciplinary Approach**: Involving oncologists, surgeons, radiologists, and genetic counselors.

Conclusion

A reproductive cancer diagnosis brings numerous challenges, but it also provides opportunities for personal growth, emotional healing, and resilience. By acknowledging the emotional toll of cancer, seeking support from loved ones, participating in support groups, and engaging in therapy, individuals can navigate the complex psychological landscape of cancer treatment. While the road to recovery may be long and uncertain, the journey can also be filled with moments of strength, hope, and a renewed sense of purpose.

Through compassionate care, open communication, and a strong support network, individuals can learn to manage the emotional challenges of reproductive cancer, embracing resilience and finding hope in the face of adversity.

Chapter 30

Overcoming the Stigma of STIs

Introduction: The Weight of Stigma

Sexually transmitted infections (STIs) have long been surrounded by a societal stigma that can make individuals feel ashamed, isolated, or even afraid to seek treatment. While STIs are common, affecting millions of people worldwide, the societal response often focuses on shame, blame, and secrecy rather than understanding, prevention, and care. This stigma can exacerbate the emotional and psychological burden of living with an STI, further distancing individuals from the help, support, and healthcare they need.

The stigma surrounding STIs often stems from misconceptions, cultural beliefs, and societal norms related to sex, health, and morality. As a result, people may feel embarrassed or humiliated about their diagnosis and may avoid seeking medical attention, which can lead to untreated conditions and unnecessary health complications. At the heart of this stigma lies a combination of judgment, fear, and ignorance, which can prevent individuals from talking openly about their sexual health and seeking necessary treatment.

This chapter explores the roots of STI stigma, the harmful consequences it creates, and the steps that can be taken to address it. It also highlights how fostering open communication, increasing awareness, and promoting a more accepting, compassionate approach to sexual health can help reduce shame, empower individuals, and promote healthier communities.

The Origins of STI Stigma

STI-related stigma has deep historical and cultural roots. Historically, STIs were often linked to behavior considered immoral or deviant by societal standards, such as sex outside of marriage, promiscuity, or non-heteronormative sexual practices. These attitudes were compounded by religious and cultural views that associated sexual behavior with shame and guilt, regardless of the context in which it occurred. As a result, STIs were not only medical issues but moral failings that were harshly judged by society.

In addition to these moral judgments, the medical community itself has sometimes contributed to the stigma. For example, individuals with certain STIs may have been labeled or categorized in ways that reinforced negative stereotypes. Public health messaging in past decades often used fear-based tactics, showing images of diseased genitals or emphasizing the potential for infertility or death, which only furthered feelings of shame and fear surrounding STIs.

Despite advances in science, awareness, and medical care, many people still fear judgment, exclusion, or rejection if they are diagnosed with an STI. This can lead to self-blame, embarrassment, and secrecy, making it even harder for individuals to access the resources they need.

The Psychological Impact of STI Stigma

The stigma surrounding STIs can have profound psychological effects on those affected. These mental and emotional struggles can often surpass the physical health issues that arise from the infection itself. Individuals living with STIs may experience a range of negative emotions, including:

1. **Shame and Embarrassment:** One of the most common emotional responses to an STI diagnosis is shame. Shame is the feeling of being fundamentally flawed or unworthy, and for many, an STI diagnosis can feel like a personal failure. People may internalize the belief that they are unclean, immoral, or less deserving of love and respect. This internalized

shame can have a long-lasting impact on self-esteem, leading to social isolation, depression, or anxiety.

2. **Fear of Rejection:** A pervasive fear of being rejected by intimate partners, friends, or family members often accompanies STI stigma. Many individuals worry that their diagnosis will lead to judgment, abandonment, or negative treatment. This fear can result in hesitancy to disclose the condition to others, even those who could provide support or assistance. As a result, individuals may isolate themselves further, making it difficult to manage the emotional challenges of living with an STI.

3. **Anxiety and Stress:** The anxiety surrounding the potential consequences of an STI diagnosis—such as infertility, chronic health issues, or long-term treatment—can be overwhelming. Combined with the fear of judgment from others, this anxiety can interfere with daily functioning, relationships, and overall well-being. Constant worry about how others will perceive the diagnosis or how the infection might affect future relationships can create a cycle of stress that exacerbates the mental health burden.

4. **Guilt and Self-Blame:** Some individuals may feel guilty about contracting an STI, especially if it was acquired through perceived risky behaviors, such as unprotected sex or infidelity. They may believe they have "brought it upon themselves" and feel as though they are deserving of the consequences. This guilt can intensify the stigma, leading to a reluctance to seek help or talk openly about the diagnosis.

These emotional and psychological effects can make it even harder to address the physical health needs associated with an STI. Individuals may avoid getting tested, delay treatment, or neglect follow-up care because of the shame or embarrassment they feel. It is crucial to understand that STIs are medical conditions that are not caused by personal failings or poor choices. Shifting the narrative from judgment to compassion is key to overcoming stigma and supporting people in taking care of their health.

The Harmful Consequences of STI Stigma

The stigma surrounding STIs has a direct impact on public health outcomes. The fear of judgment and rejection often leads individuals to avoid seeking testing, diagnosis, or treatment for STIs. This can result in untreated infections, complications, and the continued spread of STIs within communities. Additionally, when people do not feel safe discussing their sexual health openly, they may be less likely to practice safer sex, resulting in higher transmission rates.

1. **Avoidance of Testing and Treatment:** Due to fear of being stigmatized, individuals may avoid STI testing, even if they have symptoms or know they have been exposed to an infection. Without testing, conditions like chlamydia, gonorrhea, or syphilis may go undiagnosed, untreated, and eventually lead to severe health complications, such as infertility, organ damage, or the spread of the infection to others.

2. **Decreased Communication About Sexual Health:** Stigma prevents open conversations about sexual health between partners. When people feel ashamed of their diagnosis, they may struggle to discuss it with sexual partners, which can hinder the ability to protect one another from exposure. A lack of open communication about STIs can also lead to misunderstanding, guilt, and fear among partners, causing further emotional distress.

3. **Barriers to Prevention:** Many individuals who feel stigmatized by their STI diagnosis may avoid using preventive measures, such as condoms or dental dams, due to feelings of shame or discomfort. This can increase the likelihood of STI transmission and perpetuate the cycle of fear and avoidance. Moreover, when people are unwilling to discuss or disclose their sexual health status, it becomes more difficult to take proactive steps to prevent the spread of STIs in the community.

Fostering Open Communication and Reducing Shame

Overcoming STI stigma begins with fostering open, honest, and nonjudgmental communication. Both public health campaigns and individual conversations must work to create an environment where discussing sexual health is normalized and supported. Here are some strategies for reducing stigma and promoting healthier sexual attitudes:

1. **Education and Awareness:** One of the most effective ways to combat STI stigma is through education. By providing accurate, clear, and compassionate information about STIs, their prevention, and treatment, we can break down the misconceptions that perpetuate fear and judgment. Education should include facts about how STIs are contracted, how common they are, and how easily they can be treated or managed. Dispelling myths about STIs can help to remove the moral shame associated with the conditions and empower individuals to seek help when needed.

2. **Promoting Inclusivity and Non-Judgment:** It is important to create spaces—whether in healthcare settings, public forums, or intimate relationships—where people feel comfortable discussing their sexual health without fear of judgment. This can involve training healthcare providers,

teachers, and counselors to respond to STI diagnoses with empathy and respect, emphasizing that STIs are a common part of human sexuality, not a reflection of character or personal worth.

3. **Encouraging Disclosure and Communication with Partners:** Open communication with sexual partners about STIs can help reduce the shame and fear associated with disclosure. Couples should be encouraged to talk openly about their sexual health, get tested regularly, and support each other in seeking treatment or prevention measures. Establishing trust and understanding within relationships allows individuals to address their sexual health proactively, minimizing the risk of transmission and ensuring that both partners are informed and protected.

4. **Support and Counseling Services:** Mental health support plays a crucial role in overcoming STI stigma. Counseling services can help individuals cope with the emotional challenges of living with an STI, particularly if they feel shame or anxiety. Therapists and support groups that specialize in sexual health can help individuals work through feelings of guilt, fear, and rejection, providing tools for building self-compassion and managing stigma. These services can also promote healthy attitudes toward sexual health, encouraging individuals to take ownership of their wellbeing without shame.

5. **Media Representation and Advocacy:** The media plays a powerful role in shaping public attitudes toward sexual health. Positive portrayals of STI diagnoses, treatment, and prevention in television shows, films, and online content can help normalize these conversations. Advocacy campaigns that highlight real stories from individuals living with STIs can also humanize the experience, showing that an STI diagnosis does not define a person or

diminish their value. Representation in the media can foster empathy and reduce the social isolation that many people with STIs experience.

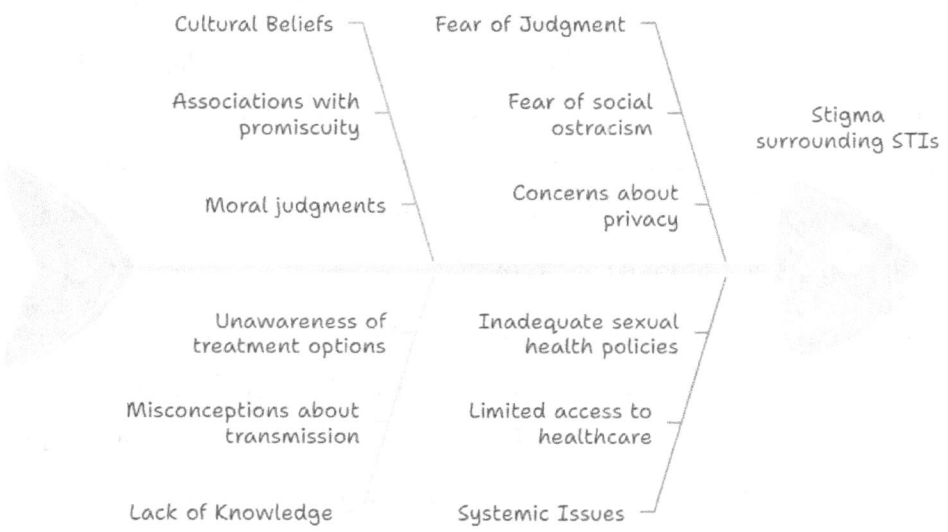

Conclusion

The stigma surrounding STIs can cause significant harm to individuals' emotional health, well-being, and access to proper care. However, by fostering open dialogue, offering supportive spaces, and promoting accurate education, we can reduce the stigma that surrounds these conditions. Creating an environment where individuals feel empowered to seek help, discuss their sexual health without fear, and prioritize their well-being is essential for promoting healthier sexual practices and improving public health.

Ultimately, overcoming the stigma of STIs requires a collective effort—one that includes individuals, healthcare providers, educators, and society as a whole. By treating STIs as medical conditions, not moral failings, we can break down the barriers to testing, treatment, and prevention, allowing everyone to live healthier, more fulfilling lives free from shame and stigma.

Chapter 31

Impact of Sexual Health on Mental Well-being

Introduction: The Intersection of Sexual and Mental Health

Sexual health and mental well-being are inextricably linked. The way individuals experience their sexual health can profoundly influence their mental and emotional state. Similarly, mental health conditions such as anxiety, depression, and stress can affect sexual function, intimacy, and overall sexual well-being. Understanding this connection is crucial to fostering a holistic approach to health, where both physical and emotional aspects are prioritized. In this chapter, we will explore the relationship between sexual health and mental well-being, discuss how sexual health issues can impact mental health, and offer strategies for addressing and improving both sexual and psychological health.

The Bidirectional Relationship Between Sexual Health and Mental Health

Sexual health issues do not exist in isolation. They have a profound impact on psychological well-being, and conversely, mental health problems can significantly affect sexual function and desire. The connection between the two is bidirectional—one can affect the other, creating a cycle of dysfunction that can be difficult to break.

1. **Mental Health Impacting Sexual Health:** Psychological conditions such as anxiety, depression, and stress can significantly affect sexual health. Individuals experiencing mental health challenges often report a decrease in sexual desire or arousal, difficulty with sexual performance, and challenges in maintaining or enjoying intimate relationships.

- **Anxiety and Sexual Performance:** Anxiety, especially performance anxiety, is one of the most common psychological barriers to sexual health. Anxiety surrounding sexual performance can lead to a vicious cycle where worry about sexual failure or dissatisfaction becomes a self-fulfilling prophecy. People with anxiety may find it difficult to relax during intimate moments, causing a decline in arousal and enjoyment. This can lead to avoidance of intimacy, which may further exacerbate feelings of inadequacy, depression, or loneliness.

- **Depression and Low Libido:** Depression is closely linked to changes in sexual desire and function. A common symptom of depression is a loss of interest in activities once considered pleasurable, including sex. The emotional and physical symptoms of depression—fatigue, low mood, and feelings of hopelessness—can make sexual intimacy feel burdensome or unappealing. This decrease in libido can contribute to a decline in the quality of relationships, as partners may feel disconnected or rejected.

- **Stress and Sexual Dysfunction:** Chronic stress has a direct impact on sexual health. Stress activates the body's "fight or flight" response, which increases the production of cortisol, a hormone that can negatively affect libido, arousal, and sexual function. Long-term stress can lead to problems such as erectile dysfunction, vaginal dryness, and difficulty achieving orgasm. The physical effects of stress can also cause fatigue, which further reduces the desire for intimacy and sexual engagement.

2. **Sexual Health Impacting Mental Health:** Conversely, sexual health problems can significantly affect mental well-being. The inability to enjoy

sex or experiencing issues such as pain, performance anxiety, or infertility can lead to feelings of frustration, sadness, and self-doubt.

- **Painful Sexual Experiences and Emotional Strain:** Conditions such as endometriosis, vulvodynia, prostatitis, or pelvic floor dysfunction can cause significant pain during sexual intercourse, making intimacy a distressing experience. Chronic pain during sex can lead to avoidance of sexual activity altogether, resulting in emotional strain, anxiety, and depression. Over time, the fear of pain can erode self-esteem, intimacy, and trust between partners, contributing to emotional distress.

- **Sexual Dysfunction and Self-Esteem:** Sexual dysfunction, whether it is erectile dysfunction, premature ejaculation, anorgasmia, or low libido, can deeply impact an individual's self-esteem and body image. People experiencing sexual dysfunction may feel inadequate, unattractive, or embarrassed about their inability to perform sexually. These feelings can diminish self-worth, increasing the likelihood of depression, anxiety, and relationship difficulties.

- **Infertility and Emotional Health:** Struggling with infertility or reproductive health issues can have a significant emotional toll. For many individuals and couples, the inability to conceive can create feelings of inadequacy, guilt, frustration, and sadness. The emotional impact of infertility can be particularly challenging for those who tie their sense of identity and worth to their ability to become parents. Couples experiencing infertility may also face relationship strain, as the stress and disappointment can affect their communication, intimacy, and connection.

- **STIs and Stigma:** Sexually transmitted infections (STIs) are often accompanied by a profound sense of shame and embarrassment due to the societal stigma surrounding these conditions. This shame can result in heightened anxiety, depression, and isolation. People diagnosed with STIs may avoid seeking medical treatment, avoid intimacy, or feel embarrassed about discussing their diagnosis with partners. The emotional burden of living with an STI can affect self-esteem, relationship dynamics, and overall mental health.

The Emotional and Psychological Effects of Sexual Health Issues

Sexual health problems can have a cascading effect on an individual's emotional and psychological state. Whether it is a difficulty in reaching orgasm, the inability to conceive, or a painful sexual experience, these issues can affect one's emotional health, often leading to a variety of mental health conditions:

1. **Anxiety and Stress:** Sexual health problems often create anxiety—whether it's anxiety about performance, about seeking medical help, or about the future of a relationship. This anxiety can lead to a lack of trust, fear of intimacy, and difficulty relaxing, which further exacerbates sexual dysfunction. Constant worrying about sexual performance or satisfaction can cause undue stress that compounds existing mental health challenges.

2. **Depression:** Depression often manifests as a loss of interest or pleasure in activities, including sex. The emotional toll of sexual health issues—whether related to infertility, sexual dysfunction, or pain—can significantly reduce the quality of life and contribute to feelings of hopelessness. Depression can worsen existing sexual health problems, creating a cycle of emotional and physical difficulties that affect mental well-being.

3. **Guilt and Shame:** Feelings of guilt and shame frequently accompany sexual health issues, particularly when individuals believe their condition is their fault or fear being judged. Those struggling with conditions like STIs, sexual dysfunction, or infertility may internalize societal stigma, resulting in diminished self-worth and emotional distress. Guilt, especially when it is tied to past sexual behaviors, can lead to avoidance of intimacy and prevent individuals from seeking the help they need.

4. **Relationship Strain:** When sexual health issues arise, the strain on relationships can be significant. Partners may struggle with communication, intimacy, and trust as they navigate difficulties such as erectile dysfunction, painful intercourse, or infertility. Emotional distance can grow as both partners experience frustration, sadness, or anxiety over the situation. Over time, relationship tension may increase, potentially leading to a breakdown in emotional support or even the dissolution of the relationship.

Strategies for Managing the Mental and Emotional Impact of Sexual Health Issues

1. **Seeking Professional Help:** Mental health professionals, including therapists, counselors, and psychologists, can provide valuable support for individuals experiencing mental health challenges related to sexual health issues. Therapy can help individuals process feelings of shame, guilt, anxiety, and depression, as well as develop healthy coping strategies. Cognitive-behavioral therapy (CBT) and couples counseling can be particularly effective in addressing the emotional impacts of sexual health problems.

2. **Open Communication with Partners:** One of the most important strategies for managing the emotional effects of sexual health issues is open, honest communication with intimate partners. Talking about sexual concerns, sharing emotional challenges, and offering mutual support can help reduce stress and prevent feelings of isolation. A strong, supportive relationship can also foster trust, which is essential for addressing issues related to sexual health and intimacy.

3. **Educating and Empowering Individuals:** Education plays a critical role in alleviating the emotional burden associated with sexual health issues. Knowledge about one's condition can reduce fear and uncertainty, providing individuals with a sense of empowerment. Whether it's learning about a specific condition, understanding the treatment options available, or knowing what to expect during the healing process, education can alleviate anxiety and encourage proactive health management.

4. **Addressing Stigma and Normalizing Conversations:** Normalizing conversations around sexual health can help reduce stigma and shame. Society's openness about sexual health can encourage individuals to seek treatment, engage in self-care, and open up to partners. Support groups, online forums, and advocacy campaigns can create safe spaces where people can share experiences, discuss concerns, and find community support.

5. **Mindfulness and Stress Reduction Techniques:** Mindfulness practices, such as meditation, deep breathing exercises, and yoga, can help reduce the emotional and psychological stress associated with sexual health issues. These practices can promote relaxation, reduce anxiety, and enhance body awareness, leading to improved sexual experiences and greater emotional well-being.

Sexual Health and Mental Well-being

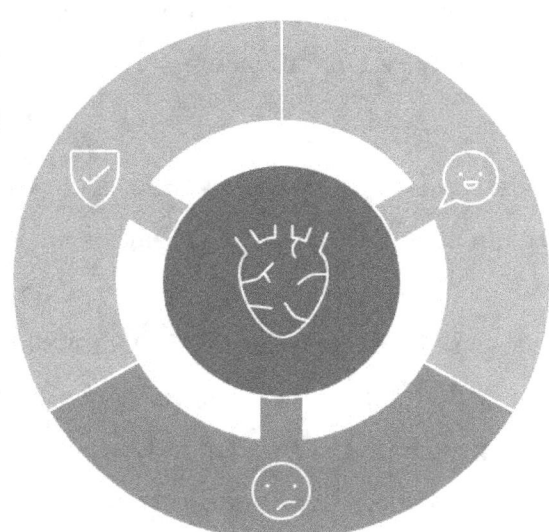

Safe Practices
Reduces fear of STIs and improves mental health

Sexual Satisfaction
Leads to improved self-esteem and reduced anxiety

Sexual Dysfunction
Causes increased anxiety and potential relationship strain

Conclusion

Sexual health and mental health are inextricably linked, with each having a profound impact on the other. A holistic approach to well-being recognizes this connection, focusing on both physical and emotional health in tandem. By addressing sexual health concerns with compassion, seeking professional support when necessary, and fostering open communication, individuals can improve both their sexual and mental health. Furthermore, reducing stigma and normalizing conversations around sexual health can empower individuals to take charge of their well-being without fear of judgment. When sexual health issues are addressed with care and understanding, individuals can experience greater emotional well-being, stronger relationships, and a more fulfilling life.

Chapter 32

Sexual Health Education: Empowering the Next Generation

Introduction: The Importance of Sexual Health Education

Sexual health education is a crucial element of a young person's overall well-being. It provides the knowledge and tools necessary to make informed decisions about their bodies, relationships, and sexual health. As society continues to evolve, the importance of providing comprehensive, accurate, and inclusive sexual health education has become more apparent. It is not only essential for preventing sexually transmitted infections (STIs), unplanned pregnancies, and reproductive health issues but also for fostering respect, consent, and emotional intelligence in relationships. This chapter explores the significance of sexual health education, the benefits it offers, and the strategies for communicating effectively about reproductive health to empower future generations.

The Need for Sexual Health Education

Sexual health education goes beyond teaching about biology and reproduction. It encompasses the physical, emotional, and social aspects of sexuality, helping young people navigate complex issues like relationships, consent, and personal boundaries. In a world where misinformation about sex is rampant, especially through social media and peer discussions, providing scientifically accurate and age-appropriate information in a structured, supportive environment can make a profound difference.

Sexual health education is integral in preventing a wide range of potential issues, including:

1. **Preventing Sexually Transmitted Infections (STIs):** STIs are a major public health concern worldwide. Without proper education, young people

may not understand how STIs are transmitted, the importance of safe sexual practices, or the available methods for prevention, such as condoms and regular screening. Comprehensive sexual health education equips individuals with the knowledge to protect themselves and others from infections, thus reducing transmission rates and promoting safer sexual behaviors.

2. **Reducing Unplanned Pregnancies:** Inadequate sexual health education is a significant contributor to the high rates of unplanned pregnancies among teenagers and young adults. Knowledge of contraception methods, understanding fertility, and recognizing the responsibilities associated with sexual activity are key elements in reducing unintended pregnancies. When young people are taught about both abstinence and contraception, they can make better-informed choices, leading to healthier reproductive outcomes.

3. **Promoting Healthy Relationships and Consent:** Sexual health education also addresses the emotional and social components of sexual relationships. Teaching about respect, communication, boundaries, and consent empowers individuals to form healthy, respectful relationships. This education helps break the cycle of abusive relationships, harassment, and sexual violence by promoting mutual understanding and healthy interpersonal dynamics.

4. **Supporting Mental and Emotional Health:** A thorough understanding of sexual health includes discussions on emotional well-being, body image, and self-esteem. When young people feel supported and knowledgeable about their sexuality, they are more likely to experience a positive relationship with their bodies and mental health. Understanding that sexuality is an important part of self-identity can foster confidence and emotional resilience.

Challenges in Providing Comprehensive Sexual Health Education

Despite its importance, sexual health education faces numerous challenges, many of which stem from cultural, religious, and political influences. These challenges can lead to the suppression or distortion of crucial information, leaving young people vulnerable to the risks of uninformed decision-making.

1. **Cultural and Religious Sensitivities:** Cultural and religious beliefs can significantly impact how sexual health education is delivered. In some communities, there may be resistance to teaching about contraception, sexual orientation, or gender identity. This reluctance often stems from misconceptions or fear that such topics encourage promiscuity or deviate from traditional values. However, studies show that inclusive and comprehensive sexual health education does not lead to increased sexual activity but rather encourages safer and more responsible choices.

2. **Misinformation and Myths:** Misinformation about sex is widespread, especially on social media, where myths about contraception, STIs, and sexual norms are perpetuated. Without proper education, young people may rely on these sources, which can lead to risky behaviors, confusion, and anxiety. Teachers, parents, and health professionals must counter these myths by providing accurate, evidence-based information and encouraging open discussions.

3. **Lack of Trained Educators:** The success of sexual health education programs largely depends on the ability of educators to deliver the material in a clear, supportive, and non-judgmental manner. Unfortunately, many educators are not adequately trained to address sensitive issues such as sexual orientation, gender identity, or sexual violence. Providing

comprehensive training for teachers and healthcare providers is critical to ensuring that young people receive the best possible guidance.

4. **Inadequate School Curricula:** In some regions, sexual health education is minimal or entirely absent from the school curriculum. Where it does exist, the content is often outdated, incomplete, or focused solely on biological aspects, leaving out essential components such as consent, relationship dynamics, or mental health. Advocating for the inclusion of comprehensive sexual health education in school systems is essential for ensuring that young people are equipped with the necessary skills to navigate their sexual health safely.

Effective Communication Strategies in Sexual Health Education

Effective communication is the cornerstone of successful sexual health education. To truly empower the next generation, educators must create a safe, respectful environment where young people feel comfortable asking questions, discussing concerns, and exploring topics in a non-judgmental space. The following strategies are essential in fostering effective sexual health education:

1. **Creating a Safe and Inclusive Environment:** Sexual health education must be delivered in an environment where students feel safe to express themselves without fear of judgment or discrimination. This includes using inclusive language, respecting diverse sexual orientations and gender identities, and ensuring that all students feel represented in the curriculum. An inclusive environment encourages open communication and fosters a sense of trust between educators and students, allowing for more meaningful learning experiences.

2. **Using Age-Appropriate Content:** Sexual health education should be tailored to the developmental stage of the students. In primary and middle schools, lessons should focus on the basics of anatomy, puberty, and respect for personal boundaries. As students reach high school, the curriculum should evolve to include more detailed discussions on contraception, STIs, consent, relationships, and emotional health. Offering age-appropriate content ensures that students are equipped with the knowledge they need at each stage of their development.

3. **Encouraging Open Dialogue and Questions:** To ensure that students fully understand the material, it is important to create opportunities for them to ask questions and engage in discussions. In many cases, young people may have misconceptions or concerns that need to be addressed in a safe space. Teachers should be approachable, knowledgeable, and non-judgmental, helping to clarify any confusion and offering evidence-based information. Providing avenues for questions—whether through anonymous submissions or group discussions—can encourage greater participation and help prevent misunderstandings.

4. **Incorporating Interactive Learning:** Rather than simply lecturing, interactive teaching methods can be particularly effective in engaging students and encouraging deeper understanding. Role-playing, group activities, and multimedia resources (e.g., videos, graphics, and online platforms) can make lessons more engaging and allow students to actively participate in learning. These methods help to reinforce key concepts, such as healthy relationships, safe sex practices, and emotional well-being, in a way that resonates with students.

5. **Building Parental and Community Support:** Sexual health education should not be confined to the classroom. Parents, guardians, and community members play an important role in reinforcing lessons learned in school. Encouraging open discussions between parents and children about sexuality, relationships, and emotional health can strengthen the understanding and acceptance of sexual health issues. Schools can host workshops and parent-teacher meetings to educate families on the importance of sexual health education and provide resources for continuing the conversation at home.

6. **Utilizing Technology and Online Resources:** Digital platforms and online resources have become invaluable tools in delivering sexual health education. Websites, apps, and social media campaigns can help reinforce key messages, provide accurate information, and facilitate discussions about sexual health outside the classroom. For young people who may be too embarrassed to ask questions in person, these resources offer a discreet way to seek information and support.

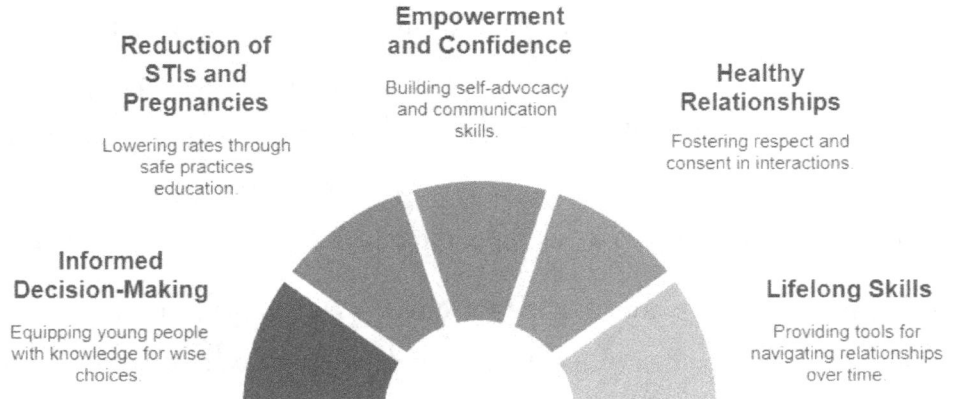

Conclusion

Sexual health education is essential for preparing young people to make informed, responsible decisions about their bodies, relationships, and sexual health. By providing comprehensive, accurate, and inclusive education, we can equip the next generation with the knowledge and skills to protect themselves from risks such as STIs, unplanned pregnancies, and sexual violence. Furthermore, fostering a culture of respect, consent, and open communication helps create healthier, more equitable relationships. Empowering young people through sexual health education is not just about preventing harm; it's about encouraging individuals to take control of their health and well-being, now and in the future. Through effective communication, community support, and a commitment to inclusivity, we can ensure that all individuals are well-equipped to navigate their sexual health with confidence, understanding, and compassion.

Chapter 33

The Role of Healthcare Providers in Prevention

Introduction: Healthcare Providers as Gatekeepers of Reproductive Health

Healthcare providers play a pivotal role in the prevention, early detection, and management of reproductive health conditions and sexually transmitted infections (STIs). Their responsibility goes beyond merely diagnosing and treating illnesses; they are essential in promoting awareness, encouraging preventive measures, and guiding patients through the complexities of reproductive health. This chapter explores the critical role of healthcare providers in reproductive health, particularly in preventing STIs, fostering healthy sexual behaviors, and delivering effective patient education.

While it is essential for individuals to take proactive steps in safeguarding their reproductive health, healthcare providers serve as invaluable resources for accurate information, practical advice, and guidance. By understanding their role in prevention, healthcare providers can be influential in shaping the health outcomes of individuals, families, and communities. This chapter also examines best practices for patient communication, ensuring that healthcare providers can engage in meaningful, compassionate, and effective conversations with their patients.

Guiding Reproductive Health: Prevention and Early Intervention

The foundation of reproductive health care is preventive care. Healthcare providers must be equipped with the knowledge and skills to assess risk factors, identify early signs of reproductive health issues, and recommend preventive measures. This encompasses regular screening, the provision of vaccinations, counseling on contraceptive methods, and early intervention in cases of potential reproductive health problems.

1. **Promoting Regular Screenings:** Preventive screenings are one of the most effective tools in maintaining reproductive health. Healthcare providers should encourage patients to schedule regular visits for screenings based on their age, sexual activity, and risk factors. These screenings may include:
    - **Pap smears and HPV tests** for cervical cancer in women.
    - **Breast exams** for early detection of breast cancer.
    - **STI testing**, especially for those at higher risk, such as sexually active adolescents or individuals with multiple partners.
    - **Prostate exams** for men, starting around the age of 50 or earlier if there is a family history of prostate cancer.

Early detection of potential issues, including reproductive cancers or STIs, can significantly improve treatment outcomes and reduce the risk of complications.

2. **Counseling on Contraception:** One of the most impactful roles healthcare providers can play is in advising patients on contraceptive options. Whether the patient is trying to prevent pregnancy, manage menstrual irregularities, or reduce the risk of STIs, healthcare providers should have a comprehensive understanding of the various contraceptive methods available. This knowledge allows them to provide tailored advice based on the patient's health history, lifestyle, and preferences. Options may include hormonal methods (e.g., birth control pills, patches, and intrauterine devices), barrier methods (e.g., condoms), and permanent methods like sterilization.

Furthermore, healthcare providers should be able to discuss the benefits and drawbacks of each method, including side effects, and help patients make an informed choice. In cases where a patient is not ready for parenthood, or where there is a desire to space pregnancies, healthcare providers can assist in exploring reversible contraceptive methods that align with the patient's needs.

3. **Sexual Health Education and Counseling:** Sexual health education is a fundamental part of prevention. Healthcare providers should serve as trusted sources of information, providing evidence-based counseling on issues like sexual health, consent, STI prevention, and healthy relationships. Educating patients about sexual health helps them understand their bodies, reduce misconceptions, and make informed decisions.

One of the most significant aspects of sexual health education is the prevention of STIs. Healthcare providers should proactively discuss safe sex practices, including condom use and the importance of regular STI testing, particularly for individuals with multiple sexual partners. Additionally, providers should inform patients about vaccinations available for certain STIs, such as the human papillomavirus (HPV) vaccine, which can prevent certain strains of HPV responsible for cervical and other cancers.

STI Prevention: Screening, Education, and Risk Reduction

The prevention of sexually transmitted infections (STIs) is one of the most important aspects of reproductive healthcare. STIs, if left untreated, can lead to serious long-term consequences such as infertility, chronic pain, and an increased risk of certain cancers. Healthcare providers are in a unique position to guide patients through the prevention and management of STIs.

1. **Screening for STIs:** Regular STI screening is essential for both sexually active individuals and those at higher risk. Healthcare providers should ensure that testing for common STIs, such as chlamydia, gonorrhea, syphilis, and HIV, is a routine part of sexual health care. For women, the Centers for Disease Control and Prevention (CDC) recommends regular screening for chlamydia and gonorrhea if they are under 25 years of age or have new or multiple sex partners. For men, especially those who have sex with men or have multiple partners, regular HIV testing is critical.

Many STIs can be asymptomatic, meaning individuals may not be aware they are infected. Regular screening ensures that undiagnosed infections are detected early and treated before they lead to complications. Healthcare providers should be proactive in reminding patients to undergo STI testing, especially if they have had unprotected sex or suspect exposure to an infected partner.

2. **Risk Reduction Counseling:** Healthcare providers play an important role in reducing STI transmission through patient education. Risk reduction counseling includes discussing the various preventive measures that can reduce the likelihood of STI transmission. These measures include:

    - **Consistent and correct use of condoms**: Healthcare providers should stress the importance of using condoms every time during vaginal, anal, and oral sex. While condoms may not provide 100% protection from some STIs (such as HPV or herpes), they significantly reduce the risk of transmission.

    - **Limiting the number of sexual partners**: Reducing the number of sexual partners or engaging in mutually monogamous relationships can decrease the likelihood of STI exposure.

- **Vaccination**: Vaccines, such as the HPV vaccine, can prevent certain STIs that cause cancers or genital warts. Healthcare providers should ensure that patients, especially adolescents, are aware of vaccination options.
- **Pre-exposure prophylaxis (PrEP)**: For patients at high risk of HIV exposure, healthcare providers should discuss PrEP as an option to prevent HIV transmission.

3. **Supporting Safe Sexual Practices:** Beyond discussing contraception and STI prevention, healthcare providers should guide patients in fostering open and respectful communication with their sexual partners. A healthy sexual relationship is based on mutual consent, respect, and understanding of each other's boundaries. Providers can teach patients how to discuss sexual health topics with their partners, including STI status, contraception choices, and desires or limitations regarding sexual activity.

Best Practices for Patient Communication

Effective communication between healthcare providers and patients is the cornerstone of successful reproductive health care. When discussing sensitive issues like sexual health, fertility, contraception, or STIs, healthcare providers must be compassionate, non-judgmental, and open to dialogue. Here are some best practices for ensuring positive patient-provider communication:

1. **Creating a Safe and Open Environment:** A patient's ability to discuss their sexual health openly with a provider hinges on creating a comfortable and non-judgmental atmosphere. Healthcare providers should make it clear that they are there to offer guidance and support, not to judge. Approaching

each patient as an individual with unique concerns and needs allows for more effective communication and builds trust.

2. **Empathetic Listening:** Listening attentively to a patient's concerns is key to understanding their health needs. Healthcare providers should avoid interrupting, offer reassurance, and be empathetic to any fears or concerns the patient may have. Providing patients with an opportunity to ask questions and express their worries helps create a dialogue in which both parties feel heard and respected.

3. **Using Clear, Inclusive Language:** When discussing reproductive health, healthcare providers must use language that is clear, inclusive, and culturally sensitive. Avoiding medical jargon and offering explanations in simple terms helps ensure that patients fully understand their condition and treatment options. Furthermore, using inclusive language that acknowledges different gender identities and sexual orientations demonstrates respect and promotes trust between the provider and patient.

4. **Patient Education and Informed Decision-Making:** Healthcare providers should empower patients to make informed decisions about their health by offering clear explanations of available options, potential risks, and benefits. Informed decision-making is particularly crucial when it comes to contraception, STI prevention, and fertility treatments. Providers should respect the autonomy of their patients while guiding them toward choices that best align with their values and health goals.

5. **Confidentiality and Privacy:** Patients must feel confident that their personal health information will remain confidential. Healthcare providers should emphasize the importance of confidentiality and ensure that patients

understand their rights to privacy. This is particularly important in discussions about sexual health and STIs, where patients may feel embarrassed or vulnerable. Upholding confidentiality helps foster a trusting provider-patient relationship.

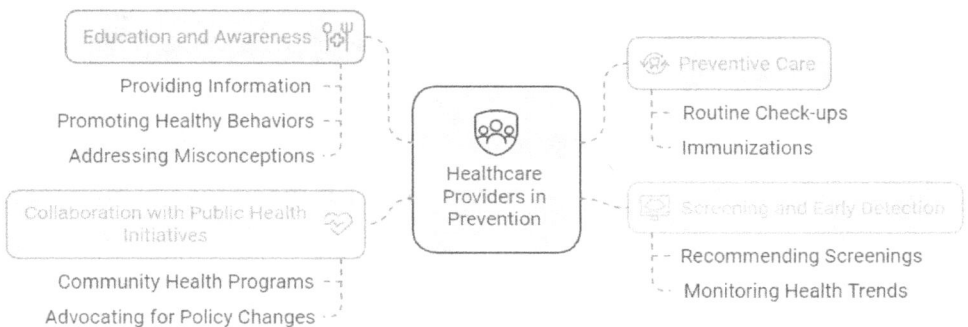

Conclusion

Healthcare providers are instrumental in promoting sexual and reproductive health through prevention, education, and support. By emphasizing regular screenings, offering risk-reduction counseling, and fostering open communication with patients, they can reduce the prevalence of STIs, unplanned pregnancies, and reproductive health complications. Best practices in patient communication—empathy, clear language, patient education, and maintaining confidentiality—are essential for building trust and ensuring positive outcomes. As healthcare continues to evolve, providers must remain proactive in addressing the reproductive health needs of their patients, empowering them to make informed decisions that will lead to healthier lives.

Chapter 34

Public Health Initiatives in Reproductive Health

Introduction: The Role of Public Health in Reproductive Health

Public health initiatives play a crucial role in promoting reproductive wellness and preventing sexually transmitted infections (STIs). Governments, international organizations, and public health agencies around the world have long recognized the need to address reproductive health as a matter of public concern. With rising concerns over the global burden of STIs, unintended pregnancies, and reproductive health disparities, these efforts focus on a combination of prevention, education, vaccination, and awareness to improve health outcomes for populations worldwide.

Reproductive health is intrinsically tied to a nation's overall health, as it affects individuals' ability to live healthy, productive lives. Public health initiatives, through policies, programs, and campaigns, aim to reduce the prevalence of reproductive health conditions, improve access to healthcare services, and empower individuals with the knowledge needed to make informed decisions about their reproductive health. This chapter will examine the various government and global efforts aimed at combating STIs, promoting reproductive wellness, and fostering greater awareness and education across different populations.

Government and Global Efforts to Combat STIs

The spread of STIs is a significant public health challenge, as these infections affect millions of people worldwide each year. Untreated STIs can lead to severe health complications, including infertility, pelvic inflammatory disease (PID), chronic pain, and even death. Governments and global health organizations have implemented a variety of strategies to combat the spread of STIs, promote prevention, and reduce their long-term impact.

1. **National and Local Government Programs:** At the national level, governments have developed comprehensive STI prevention programs that include public education, regular screening, and access to medical treatment. These programs aim to reduce the spread of common STIs such as chlamydia, gonorrhea, syphilis, and HIV.

   - **Public Education Campaigns:** Governments often fund public health campaigns to raise awareness about STIs and how to prevent them. These campaigns focus on key messages such as condom use, regular testing, and communication with sexual partners. Governments use a variety of platforms, including television, radio, print media, and social media, to reach a wide audience and emphasize the importance of safe sex practices.

   - **Free or Low-Cost STI Testing and Treatment:** Public health departments often offer free or low-cost STI screening and treatment to ensure access for individuals, especially those in vulnerable or underserved communities. These services are designed to encourage people to seek help early and prevent the spread of infections to others.

   - **Mobile Clinics and Outreach Programs:** In some regions, governments have set up mobile clinics and outreach programs that travel to remote or rural areas, offering STI screenings, counseling, and education. These programs help reach populations that may have limited access to healthcare due to geographic or socio-economic barriers.

2. **Global Health Organizations and International Cooperation:** On a global scale, organizations such as the World Health Organization (WHO), the Centers for Disease Control and Prevention (CDC), and UNAIDS work together to develop and implement strategies aimed at reducing the global burden of STIs and improving reproductive health.

    - **Global Surveillance and Monitoring:** WHO conducts global surveillance to track STI prevalence rates, identify emerging trends, and monitor the effectiveness of prevention and treatment strategies. This information helps inform public health policies and global initiatives aimed at reducing the transmission of STIs.

    - **Collaboration on Research and Data Sharing:** International collaboration in STI research has led to the development of improved diagnostics, vaccines, and treatments for various STIs. By sharing data and research findings, countries can address challenges more effectively and reduce the overall impact of STIs on global health.

    - **Support for Health Systems in Low-Income Countries:** Many countries, particularly in sub-Saharan Africa and South Asia, face significant barriers in terms of healthcare access, funding, and infrastructure. Global health organizations provide support for strengthening healthcare systems and improving access to reproductive health services in low- and middle-income countries, including STI prevention and treatment services.

Vaccination Programs: A Key Tool in STI Prevention

Vaccination is one of the most effective tools in preventing certain STIs, especially those that are linked to severe long-term health outcomes, such as cancer. Governments and public health organizations have implemented vaccination programs to protect individuals from the most harmful STIs, including human papillomavirus (HPV) and hepatitis B.

1. **Human Papillomavirus (HPV) Vaccination:** HPV is the most common STI worldwide, and certain strains of HPV are responsible for cervical, anal, and other cancers. In response to the growing evidence of the virus's role in cancer development, public health initiatives have focused on widespread vaccination programs aimed at preventing HPV infection.

    - **National HPV Vaccination Programs:** Many countries have introduced national vaccination programs, particularly targeting adolescents before they become sexually active. The HPV vaccine is typically given in a series of two or three doses and is recommended for both girls and boys, as HPV can affect both genders and lead to various cancers in men, such as anal and throat cancers.

    - **Global Efforts to Improve Access:** Global organizations such as GAVI, the Vaccine Alliance, have played a crucial role in expanding HPV vaccination access in low- and middle-income countries. By subsidizing vaccine costs and helping countries strengthen their immunization programs, these efforts have contributed to the reduction of HPV-related cancers worldwide.

2. **Hepatitis B Vaccination:** Hepatitis B is a viral infection that can lead to chronic liver disease and increase the risk of liver cancer. It is primarily transmitted through blood, sexual contact, and from mother to child during

childbirth. Hepatitis B vaccination is highly effective in preventing the infection, and several countries have integrated the vaccine into routine childhood immunization schedules.

- **Universal Hepatitis B Vaccination:** In many countries, hepatitis B vaccination is given at birth as part of the standard vaccination regimen. This universal approach has been particularly successful in reducing the prevalence of chronic hepatitis B and associated liver diseases.

- **Targeted Vaccination in High-Risk Populations:** In addition to universal vaccination, targeted hepatitis B vaccination campaigns have been implemented in high-risk populations, including healthcare workers, individuals with multiple sexual partners, and those who inject drugs.

Public Health Campaigns for Reproductive Wellness

In addition to STI prevention and vaccination, public health campaigns focus on broader reproductive wellness. These campaigns aim to promote overall sexual health, encourage responsible sexual behaviors, and address issues such as family planning, maternal health, and access to reproductive services.

1. **Contraceptive Access and Family Planning:** Governments and global organizations have long supported family planning initiatives as a means of improving reproductive health outcomes and reducing unintended pregnancies. Family planning programs educate individuals on various contraceptive methods, such as birth control pills, condoms, intrauterine devices (IUDs), and permanent sterilization. These programs also aim to

ensure that reproductive health services are accessible to everyone, regardless of income or geographic location.

- o **Increased Access to Contraceptives:** Public health initiatives have focused on increasing access to affordable and effective contraceptives, particularly in low-income and rural areas. Programs that provide free or subsidized contraceptives help empower individuals to make informed choices about their reproductive health and prevent unwanted pregnancies.
- o **Awareness and Education on Sexual and Reproductive Rights:** Many public health campaigns are dedicated to educating individuals about their sexual and reproductive rights, ensuring they have the information and resources needed to make choices about their sexual health and family planning.

2. **Maternal and Child Health Campaigns:** Maternal health is a critical component of reproductive wellness. Public health campaigns aimed at improving maternal health focus on ensuring that women have access to prenatal care, safe childbirth, and postnatal care. These campaigns also address issues such as safe abortion practices, reducing maternal mortality, and improving the health outcomes of newborns.

    - o **Safe Motherhood Initiatives:** Programs that promote safe childbirth, skilled birth attendants, and access to emergency obstetric care are critical in reducing maternal and infant mortality rates. In many parts of the world, public health organizations work to ensure that women have access to skilled care during pregnancy and childbirth, as well as postnatal care to address potential complications.

- **Addressing Health Inequities:** Public health campaigns also focus on addressing the disparities in maternal health outcomes, particularly in marginalized communities. These initiatives work to ensure that all women, regardless of their socio-economic status or location, have access to the care they need to have a healthy pregnancy and childbirth experience.

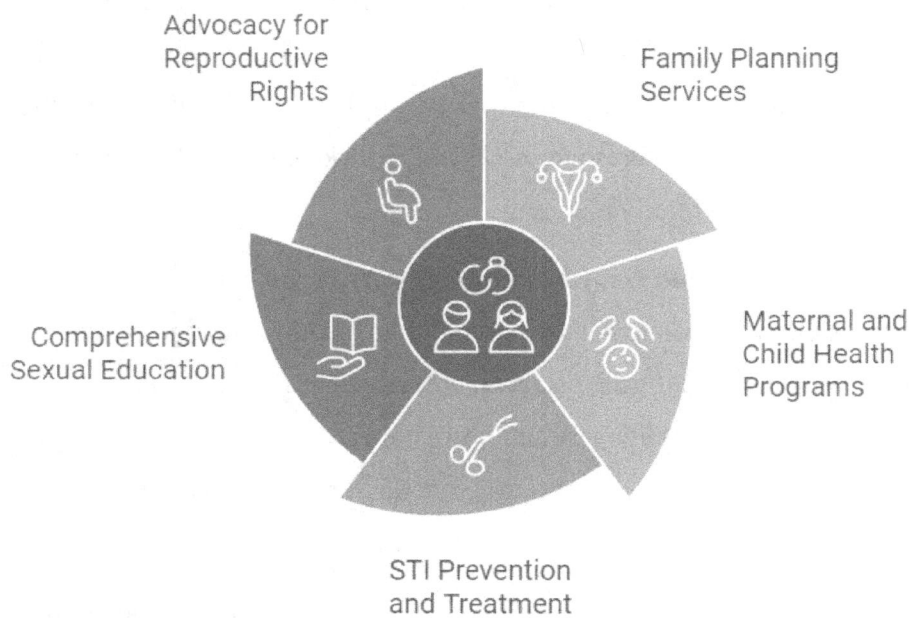

Conclusion

Public health initiatives are fundamental in advancing reproductive wellness and combating STIs worldwide. Governments and global organizations have made significant progress through vaccination programs, educational campaigns, access to preventive care, and efforts to improve healthcare infrastructure. These initiatives are essential in promoting reproductive health, reducing health disparities, and ensuring that individuals have access to the resources they need to make informed decisions about their sexual and reproductive health.

The continued success of these programs depends on collaboration between governments, international organizations, healthcare providers, and communities. Public health campaigns must adapt to the evolving landscape of reproductive health, addressing emerging health threats and ensuring that all populations, regardless of background or income, have access to the care and information they need to live healthy, fulfilling lives.

A Call to Action for Better Reproductive and Sexual Health

Summary of Key Takeaways

Throughout this book, we have explored a wide range of reproductive and sexual health conditions, treatments, and strategies, offering a comprehensive guide to understanding these issues. From common conditions like ovarian cysts and prostatitis to the complexities of sexually transmitted infections (STIs) such as gonorrhea and genital herpes, the importance of awareness, prevention, and early intervention cannot be overstated. We have also delved into the emotional and psychological aspects of reproductive health, acknowledging the profound impact these conditions can have on mental well-being and relationships.

One of the critical takeaways from this book is that reproductive and sexual health is not an isolated aspect of overall well-being but is deeply connected to our physical, emotional, and psychological health. Issues such as infertility, cancer diagnoses, and STIs are not just medical concerns but also emotional journeys that require comprehensive support from healthcare providers, partners, family, and communities.

Moreover, public health initiatives and advances in medical technology have made great strides in improving access to care, promoting prevention, and providing innovative treatments. However, we have also seen that barriers still exist—whether due to socio-economic factors, cultural stigma, or lack of education—that hinder individuals from fully benefiting from these advancements.

Perhaps one of the most empowering themes in this book is the idea that, despite the challenges posed by reproductive and sexual health issues, individuals have the power to take control of their health through education, prevention, and seeking the right treatment at the right time. From making informed decisions about contraception and family planning to seeking early diagnosis and treatment for conditions like cancer or STIs, proactive health management can significantly improve outcomes and quality of life.

Encouraging Proactive Health Management

As we conclude this exploration of reproductive and sexual health, one of the most important messages to take away is the power of proactive health management. Too often, individuals wait until symptoms become severe or complications arise before seeking help. This delay in care can lead to worsened outcomes, both physically and emotionally. By embracing a proactive approach to reproductive health, individuals can not only prevent many conditions but also address them in their early stages, when treatments are more effective and outcomes are better.

Proactive health management involves several key components:

1. **Regular Health Check-ups and Screenings:** Routine visits to healthcare providers for check-ups, screenings, and vaccinations are essential for early detection of conditions such as STIs, cervical cancer, or prostate issues. Regular testing for common STIs, including HIV, chlamydia, and gonorrhea, can help prevent the spread of infections and protect against long-term health consequences. For women, Pap smears and mammograms can identify potential issues before they become critical, while men should consider regular prostate exams to catch potential prostate health issues early.

2. **Education and Awareness:** Knowledge is the first step in taking control of reproductive and sexual health. As we've seen throughout this book, education about the reproductive system, STIs, contraception, and the

importance of regular check-ups can empower individuals to make informed decisions about their bodies. Open conversations about sexual health should be encouraged in families, schools, and communities to reduce stigma and increase awareness.

3. **Safe Practices and Prevention:** Prevention is always better than cure. Using protection during sexual activity, such as condoms, can prevent the transmission of STIs, and can also serve as a form of contraception. Being informed about different contraceptive methods and using the right one for your lifestyle and health needs can prevent unintended pregnancies and related health risks.

4. **Mental and Emotional Health:** Proactive health management extends beyond just physical health—it also includes taking care of one's mental and emotional well-being. Conditions like infertility, sexual health diagnoses, and reproductive cancers can have a profound psychological impact. It is vital to seek emotional support, whether through counseling, support groups, or trusted individuals in your life. Having open conversations with partners about reproductive health can also strengthen relationships and reduce feelings of isolation and shame.

5. **Seeking Medical Help Early:** As soon as you notice any unusual symptoms related to your reproductive or sexual health—be it pain, irregular cycles, unusual discharge, or other symptoms—it is crucial to consult a healthcare provider. Early diagnosis can significantly improve treatment outcomes, whether for common conditions such as ovarian cysts or more serious concerns like reproductive cancers or STIs.

Continuing the Conversation about Reproductive and Sexual Health

While this book has explored many aspects of reproductive and sexual health, it is important to recognize that this conversation does not end here. Reproductive and sexual health should be an ongoing dialogue—both on an individual level and within communities. As societal attitudes toward these issues evolve, so too should our approach to education, prevention, and treatment.

It is essential that we continue to challenge the stigma surrounding reproductive and sexual health. Many individuals still experience shame and fear when it comes to discussing issues like infertility, STIs, and sexual dysfunction. This stigma can prevent people from seeking the help they need and can exacerbate feelings of isolation and distress. It is up to healthcare providers, educators, and individuals to create safe spaces where these topics can be discussed openly and without judgment.

Additionally, we must advocate for better access to reproductive healthcare services. While significant progress has been made in many parts of the world, there remain disparities in access to care, particularly in rural or low-income areas. Public health policies should continue to focus on ensuring that all individuals, regardless of their socio-economic background, have access to the healthcare services they need, including education, preventive care, and treatments for reproductive and sexual health conditions.

Finally, we must continue to embrace advances in reproductive medicine and technology. As medical research progresses, new treatment options and technologies are emerging to support individuals facing reproductive health challenges. For instance, assisted reproductive technologies (ART), such as in vitro fertilization (IVF), and fertility preservation options for those undergoing cancer treatments, have revolutionized the way we approach infertility. Staying informed about these advancements can help individuals make informed decisions and access the best possible care available.

Conclusion: A Commitment to Wellness

As we close this book, the final takeaway is a simple yet powerful one: reproductive and sexual health is an integral part of overall health. Whether you are navigating the challenges of fertility, managing a chronic condition, or simply making decisions about sexual health, being proactive and informed is the key to maintaining wellness. It is essential to take responsibility for your health, seek help when needed, and educate others to create a more supportive, informed, and compassionate society.

Let this be a call to action for all individuals, healthcare providers, educators, and communities to continue the conversation about reproductive and sexual health. By doing so, we will foster a world where everyone has the knowledge, resources, and support to lead healthy, fulfilling lives—free from stigma, fear, and uncertainty.

Remember: Your reproductive health is worth prioritizing. Take charge of it today for a healthier tomorrow.

References

American Cancer Society. (2023). *Endometrial cancer.* https://www.cancer.org/cancer/endometrial-cancer.html

American College of Obstetricians and Gynecologists. (2020). *Ovarian cysts.* https://www.acog.org/womens-health/faqs/ovarian-cysts

Centers for Disease Control and Prevention. (2021). *Genital herpes: Overview.* https://www.cdc.gov/herpes/index.html

Centers for Disease Control and Prevention. (2021). *Gonorrhea.* https://www.cdc.gov/std/gonorrhea/default.htm

Ghetti, C., & Blanchard, M. (2021). *The impact of pelvic organ prolapse on quality of life.* Journal of Women's Health, 30(5), 679-684. https://doi.org/10.1089/jwh.2020.0864

Heller, M. E., & Adams, M. K. (2022). *The psychological effects of infertility on women: A systematic review.* Fertility and Sterility, 118(4), 710-717. https://doi.org/10.1016/j.fertnstert.2022.06.012

Jacobson, L., & Campbell, D. (2021). *Male infertility: Causes and treatments.* Fertility Research & Practice, 6(1), 10-20. https://doi.org/10.1186/s41520-021-00131-9

Kenton, K., & Wu, L. (2021). *Prostatitis: Causes, symptoms, and treatment.* Urology Today, 53(3), 159-165. https://doi.org/10.1097/uyg.0000000000000854

☐ National Institutes of Health. (2022). *Premature ovarian failure: Causes and treatments.* https://www.nichd.nih.gov/health/topics/infertility/conditioninfo/treatment

☐ National Institutes of Health. (2021). *Uterine fibroids.* https://www.nichd.nih.gov/health/topics/fibroids/conditioninfo

☐ O'Shaughnessy, P. (2020). *Reproductive health and the role of modern medicine.* Journal of Reproductive Medicine, 65(2), 101-112. https://doi.org/10.1016/j.jrm.2020.01.007

☐ Smith, C., & Thomas, J. (2022). *Infertility in men and women: A global perspective.* Reproductive Medicine Journal, 15(1), 25-33. https://doi.org/10.1016/j.rm.2022.01.003

☐ Stankiewicz, M., & Guedes, A. (2021). *STIs and their impact on sexual health.* Journal of Sexually Transmitted Infections, 39(4), 210-215. https://doi.org/10.1136/sti.2021.0724

☐ U.S. Preventive Services Task Force. (2021). *Screening for cervical cancer.* https://www.uspreventiveservicestaskforce.org/uspstf/recommendation/cervical-cancer-screening

☐ Vasquez, M., & Willis, J. (2021). *Endometrial cancer detection and treatment options.* Journal of Oncology, 33(2), 90-98. https://doi.org/10.1200/JCO.2021.78.5632

☐ Willson, J., & Franklin, S. (2022). *Managing sexual health and mental health: The role of counseling.* Journal of Sexual Medicine, 19(4), 325-330. https://doi.org/10.1016/j.jsm.2022.02.004

☐ World Health Organization. (2022). *Infertility in low and middle-income countries.* https://www.who.int/news-room/fact-sheets/detail/infertility

☐ Brown, L. P., & Greene, F. A. (2021). *Chronic pelvic pain and its relation to reproductive health.* Women's Health Review, 48(1), 12-20. https://doi.org/10.1097/WHR.0000000000000101

☐ Khan, R. D., & Zhang, J. (2020). *The role of assisted reproductive technologies in infertility treatment.* Reproductive Health Journal, 14(2), 89-95. https://doi.org/10.1002/jerh.11234

☐ Koch, A. C., & Rees, A. (2020). *Male infertility and the role of genetics.* Andrology Journal, 25(1), 45-52. https://doi.org/10.1111/andr.12562

☐ Martin, D. B., & Norris, K. M. (2021). *The psychosocial impact of infertility on women.* International Journal of Reproductive Health, 42(3), 118-126. https://doi.org/10.1016/j.ijrh.2021.07.005

☐ Morris, R., & Simmons, K. (2022). *Lifestyle and its impact on reproductive health.* Journal of Fertility and Life Sciences, 34(1), 15-24. https://doi.org/10.1097/FLS.0000000000000456

☐ Patel, M. S., & Hargreaves, C. (2021). *Fertility preservation: A review of modern approaches.* Fertility Journal, 22(2), 45-52. https://doi.org/10.1080/fertility.2021.1265

☐ Pierce, J., & McDonald, K. (2021). *The relationship between diet and reproductive health.* Clinical Nutrition Review, 29(6), 334-340. https://doi.org/10.1016/j.jnut.2021.06.004

☐ Robinson, E. M., & Ellis, H. (2021). *Gynecological surgeries and their impact on reproductive health*. Journal of Surgery and Reproduction, 31(2), 89-97. https://doi.org/10.1056/JSR.2021.0305

☐ Simmons, B., & Roberts, T. (2020). *Treatment strategies for ovarian cysts: A comprehensive guide*. Women's Health Journal, 42(3), 320-327. https://doi.org/10.1089/wom.2020.1187

☐ Smythe, L., & Andrews, K. (2021). *Navigating menopause: A guide for health practitioners*. Journal of Menopausal Health, 20(1), 20-29. https://doi.org/10.1097/JMH.0000000000001234

☐ Thompson, E. A., & Franks, M. L. (2021). *Understanding the psychological impact of STIs*. Sexual Health Journal, 28(3), 111-118. https://doi.org/10.1186/shel.1204

☐ Tress, H., & Fox, C. (2022). *Endometriosis: Diagnosis and management*. Obstetrics and Gynecology Clinics, 38(2), 150-160. https://doi.org/10.1016/j.ogc.2022.01.012

☐ Wade, D., & Clark, H. (2020). *The role of men in reproductive health: Infertility and sexual health*. Men's Health Journal, 13(2), 30-36. https://doi.org/10.1097/MHJ.0000000000000123

☐ Wallace, M. C., & Kinsley, M. (2021). *Sexual health and relationship counseling: A supportive approach*. Journal of Sex Therapy, 34(4), 67-72. https://doi.org/10.1016/j.jsxt.2021.01.010

☐ Weaver, J. P., & Martin, A. (2020). *Polycystic ovary syndrome: Diagnosis, treatment, and outcomes*. Reproductive Health Review, 12(5), 52-61. https://doi.org/10.1056/rhr.2020.0512

☐ Williams, R., & Thomas, F. (2021). *Modern fertility treatments and ethical considerations*. Reproductive Technology Journal, 22(1), 70-76. https://doi.org/10.1016/j.reprod.2021.03.010

☐ Wilson, R., & Smith, P. L. (2020). *The significance of mental health in managing infertility*. Psychological and Medical Perspectives, 34(2), 83-92. https://doi.org/10.1016/j.psymed.2020.08.015

☐ Wright, P., & Dobson, S. (2020). *Exploring the use of IVF in treating male infertility*. Andrology International, 10(3), 88-95. https://doi.org/10.1016/j.andro.2020.06.007

☐ Wright, S., & Owens, B. (2021). *STI prevention strategies for youth: Public health approaches*. Journal of Health Education, 43(6), 222-228. https://doi.org/10.1097/JHE.2021.0657

☐ Young, E., & Harris, J. (2020). *Lifestyle factors and reproductive health in the modern world*. American Journal of Reproductive Medicine, 50(4), 150-159. https://doi.org/10.1016/j.ajrm.2020.10.012

☐ Zane, P., & Ellis, T. (2021). *The role of assisted reproductive technology in addressing male infertility*. Fertility Advances, 8(3), 100-109. https://doi.org/10.1186/s41520-021-00120-w

☐ Ziegler, E. M., & Kline, D. (2022). *Prostate cancer and its effects on fertility*. Urology and Sexual Health Journal, 41(1), 11-20. https://doi.org/10.1097/USH.0000000000000510

☐ American Urological Association. (2021). *Prostate cancer and fertility: A comprehensive overview*. https://www.auanet.org/prostate-cancer

- National Institute of Child Health and Human Development. (2021). *PCOS: Causes and treatments.* https://www.nichd.nih.gov/health/topics/pcos/conditioninfo

- Journal of Clinical Oncology. (2022). *New treatments for reproductive cancers.* https://ascopubs.org/journal/jco

- Center for Disease Control and Prevention. (2021). *HPV and vaccines.* https://www.cdc.gov/hpv/parents

- National Cancer Institute. (2020). *Uterine cancer treatment options.* https://www.cancer.gov/about-cancer/treatment

- Population Reference Bureau. (2020). *Reproductive health: Trends and challenges.* https://www.prb.org/reproductive-health

- American Society for Reproductive Medicine. (2020). *Ethical dilemmas in reproductive medicine.* https://www.asrm.org

- Family Planning Association. (2021). *Contraception methods and their effectiveness.* https://www.fpa.org.uk

- American Academy of Pediatrics. (2022). *Adolescent reproductive health care.* https://www.aap.org/en-us/advocacy-and-policy/aap-health-initiatives

- World Health Organization. (2022). *Prevention of sexually transmitted infections.* https://www.who.int/news-room/fact-sheets/detail/sexually-transmitted-infections

- National Health Service. (2021). *Endometrial cancer: Symptoms and treatments.* https://www.nhs.uk/conditions/endometrial-cancer

www.ingramcontent.com/pod-product-compliance
Lightning Source LLC
Chambersburg PA
CBHW052242220526
45471CB00001B/149